TAKING YOUR BACK
TO THE FUTURE

How to get a pain-free back and
total health with chiropractic care

by W. MICHAEL GAZDAR, D.C., C.C.S.P.
Doctor of Chiropractic
Certified Chiropractic Sports Physician

Published by John Muir Chiropractic Center

Published and distributed by
John Muir Chiropractic Center
1776 Ygnacio Valley Road, Suite 201
Walnut Creek, California 94598
phone: (925) 939-1738
fax: (925) 939-8017
email: michael@gazdar.com
web: www.gazdar.com

Cover design by Marty Rollinson and Hamid Sadeghi.
All photos by Hamid Sadeghi unless otherwise noted.
Preparation for 2nd printing by The Courtenay Design Group.

Library of Congress Catalog Card Number: 95-75676
Gazdar, Michael

TAKING YOUR BACK TO THE FUTURE: How to
get a pain-free back and total health with chiropractic care

ISBN 0-9645301-1-2 Trade Paper Edition

Printed in the United States of America

③4 5 6 7 8 9 10

DEDICATION

A doctor and teacher has to learn many things from many different people. I want to dedicate this book to the three closest people in my life; each has loved and taught me in a unique way.

First, my mother was my earliest teacher and has always believed in me, no matter what I did. Her love has never wavered. Second, my wife Teri has been my second teacher. She taught me about life and how to love unconditionally and unselfishly. Third, my sons—Christian Michael has been my greatest teacher and Brandon Michael the renewed light in my life. They have taught me more about myself in the short time I've known them than I could ever imagine. As with my mother and wife, their love is without question or condition.

I have also had professional teachers to whom I would like to make this special dedication. Dr. Daniel Murphy has been my chiropractic mentor since my start at chiropractic college. He was my first chiropractor and helped cure my asthma; he also made me believe.

Dr. Michael Schmidt has been a teacher and personal friend of mine for many years. Along with Dan Murphy he was the first to encourage me to teach chiropractic as well as practice it. Each has set the example that you must give back to the profession which has given you so much.

Dr. Don Harrison and Dr. Sang Harrison have been instrumental in founding and developing the best chiropractic technique in the discipline.

Fourth, Dr. Gerard Clum, President of Life Chiropractic College West, has consistently led our profession to new heights from San Lorenzo, California to Washington, DC. Dr. Clum will stop at nothing to get the truth about chiropractic to the ears and hearts of the people of the world.

Fifth, Dr. Sid Williams, founder of Life Chiropractic College in Georgia, had the dream for Life Chiropractic College West in

California. Dr. Williams has helped spread the word of chiropractic around the world in his relentless quest to help people stay healthy without the use of drugs or surgery.

All my patients have taught me how to be a "real doctor" while my students at Life Chiropractic College West have been, are now and will always be my best instructors.

ACKNOWLEDGEMENTS

This book would not be here without the talents of some very special people. I believed it would take about six months from the time I started writing this book until it appeared on the shelves of your friendly neighborhood bookstore. Was I wrong! There are so many people I need to thank that it would take a complete book to thank them all. If I inadvertently omit you, please forgive me and call me before the next edition comes out.

Many old and new friends and colleagues have helped me. Hamid Sadeghi has been my art director, photographer, encourager and friend. He knew nothing about chiropractic but jumped right in and became my strongest supporter. Larry and Linda Wyner have contributed constant effort, consistently great editorial suggestions, and encouragement to help make this book what it has become. Marty Rollinson has helped design a great book cover and Mae Schoenig has provided the wonderful graphics. Jerry G. Wright, Esq. has been a great attorney. Thanks to my first editor three years ago, Deborah Fields. The final project has changed, but your early suggestions were of great value. Thanks also to Jacqueline Teele, who did a beautiful job merging text and pictures into what you see here.

The following people know how much they have helped me; I thank you all. Dr. Adi Adins, Marian Adins, Andrea Adins, Lizzy Adins, Togo Yoshioka, Elaine Yoshioka, Mike Yoshioka,

MikeyYoshioka, Jade Yoshioka, Dale Lineaweaver, Dr. David Amaral, Dr. Ronald Fritz, Dr. Darrell Lavin, Dr. Charles Ward, Dr. Kirby Landis, Dr. Patricia Gayman, Dr. Jim Parker, Dr. Craig Johnson, Dr. Malik Slosberg, Dr. Mark Victor Hansen, Dr. Franco Columbu, Dr. Tom Deters, former international model Jill (Van Doren) Totten, former University of Washington and All American hurdler Claudine Robinson, Dave Perman, Michael Rath, Camran, Leila and Beatrice Sadeghi, Barbara Delli Gatti, Wanda Butterly and everyone at Life Chiropractic College West Library, Celia Kaplan, Debbie Martin, Debbie Fisher, Debbie Palmer, Michael Sike, Sharyn Abbott, Fred Schultz, Dr. Anthony Roberts, Dr. Jeffrey Lant, Dr. Ethan Feldman, Dean Diltz, Larry Turetski, Dr. Lou Solis, Kathy, Peggy and Julie at Mark Victor Hansen's office, Michael Potter, Marcell Saba, Janet DeJesus, Linda Henry, Lisa Clark and Michelle Ogata at Muscle and Fitness, Kurt Rogers and Edvins Beitiks at the San Francisco Examiner, cartoonists Garry Trudeau and Tom Meyer, Carla Stiff and Marty at Universal Press Syndicate, Theresa Crouch at U.M.I., Jackie Jones at the San Francisco Chronicle, Barbara Blum and Anna Duckworth at KCBS radio in San Francisco, Rob Cook at Courtenay Design, Miles, Scott and Mansoor at Cat's Pajamas, Glenda at Palmer College, Dave Gallegos, Dr. Steve Albrect, Ms. Suzanne Ray, Mr. Jim Hawkins, Dr. James Konlande, Drs. Charisse and Ronald Desmarais, Dr. Patrick and Linda Hickman, Thom Parrino, Laura Niznik, Leonard and Denise Nelson, Dr. Dennis Nikitow, Dr. Shakati Singh Khalsa, Dr. Linda Rhodes, my anonymous patients who let me use their x-rays and stories, and finally my models Smokey, Snoflake and Garfield.

In Memorial

This page is in memory of Daniel Reid, M.D. and his wife Barbara who died in early September, 1991. Dr. Reid was an excellent heart surgeon, mountain climber, polo player and general sportsman. He and his wife were on the first American team to scale the east side of Mt. Everest in 1983. Dan made it to the summit while Barbara operated the base camps. They died on Mt. Kenya in Africa in bad weather by a fall sometime during the night. Dan was a good friend to everyone he met, from cowboys to surgeons, including this author. He was the first to applaud my decision to become a chiropractor instead of a medical doctor. We miss you, Dan.

DISCLAIMER

This book is intended primarily for the person who knows little, if anything, about chiropractic and wishes to learn about this valuable form of health care. It is not meant to be a textbook; however, there are some technical references presented which are too important to omit. These have been included in the endnotes for further research if you wish. All of the stories cited are real, although most of the names have been changed to protect the patients' identities and dignity. You should not try to diagnose yourself or use any of the therapies presented here without the advice and/or supervision of your chiropractor. Finally, you should go only to a licensed, Board-approved Doctor of Chiropractic for care. Any treatment regimes are between you and your doctor. Neither the author nor publisher can be held liable for any therapies rendered.

NOTE

The models depicted in this book are wearing exercise outfits to better illustrate the anatomy of the body. Many chiropractic techniques allow you to stay fully clothed during your office visit.

TABLE OF CONTENTS

TABLE OF CONTENTS IN DETAIL

FOREWORD

by Dr. Mark Victor Hansen

At no time in our history has the lay-person been so assertive in questioning the DOCTOR. We are at the crossroads of a great medical revolution. People are not only questioning, they are demanding truthful answers. They are no longer willing to leave everything up to the "expert" where their health is concerned.

I have been a chiropractic patient for many years. I have seen to it that my wife gets her back checked and adjusted weekly and our two beautiful daughters have gotten regular spinal check-ups from birth. I have dedicated much of my yearly speaking schedule to chiropractic groups and their patients, and I feel a special affinity for my chiropractic "family."

There is a great deal of misconception about chiropractic care. Dr. Michael Gazdar has written a wonderful book which will challenge many of the ideas you have about health. He points out that while medicine tends to go aggressively after the symptoms after you have become sick, chiropractic focuses on a gentle, natural return to health. And it keeps you there! All the healing takes place without the use of drugs or surgery.

While many know that chiropractors can fix a bad back, few realize there have been thousands of cases of serious "medical" diseases resolved under chiropractic care. Dr. Gazdar gives you the stories and also provides the research showing why asthma, diabetes, hypertension and other health challenges respond to this ancient, drugless approach.

This is a situation where everyone is better off for having read this book and no one is worse off. There is something here for everyone: a rationale for seeking out a chiropractor, how to find a good chiropractor, different techniques, helpful back exercises and more.

I have said that all leaders in society are readers, but not all readers are leaders. It is my fervent hope and ardent desire that you become a leader when it comes to you and your family's health. This book is a *wow*!

Here's wishing you abundant health!

Chiropractic care

needs no special tools.

It puts nothing into the body

and takes nothing out.

PREFACE

by Dr. Gerard Clum,
President, Life Chiropractic College West

For many, understanding the relationship of chiropractic care to back pain is a logical and reasonable conclusion. But for persons who have experienced the sometimes very dramatic effects of spinal adjusting on health problems apparently far removed from the spine, the low back pain conclusion is quite incomplete. Attempting to relate the greater context of chiropractic care to the health care consumer is one of the greatest challenges that faces every doctor of chiropractic.

Dr. Michael Gazdar offers the chiropractic provider and patient alike a great service relative to understanding the concepts that underlie chiropractic care. Through his presentation you have the opportunity to better understand the elements that may most likely combine to create a state of optimum health. You will also understand that your health care is fundamentally your responsibility. You will also learn what resources your doctor of chiropractic brings to bear on your behalf.

Health care is in a state of great change. We are examining how we receive our health care, from whom we receive our health care, how we pay for our health care and most importantly, what health care interventions help us and with what consequences. This last area is one where you will see some big surprises in the years to come. Many of the standard medical approaches to health care will be discarded and less invasive, more natural approaches that rely on the body's own inborn ability to heal will be utilized. Chiropractic care will undoubtedly become one of the standard components of our health care system. Your concern for your health and the health of your loved ones is truly commendable. Understanding the concepts and ideas presented in *Taking Your Back To The Future* will enable you to be a more active participant in your health care and will help assure that you will have the opportunity to add life to your years and years to your life!

"First, a new theory is attacked as absurd, then it is admitted to be true, but obvious and insignificant; finally it is seen to be so important that its adversaries claim that they themselves discovered it."

William James

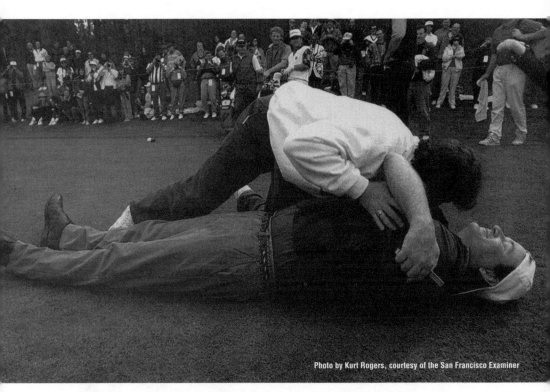

Photo by Kurt Rogers, courtesy of the San Francisco Examiner

The author adjusting actor Bill Murray at the 1994 AT&T Golf Tournament at Spyglass Hills Golf Course on the seventh tee.

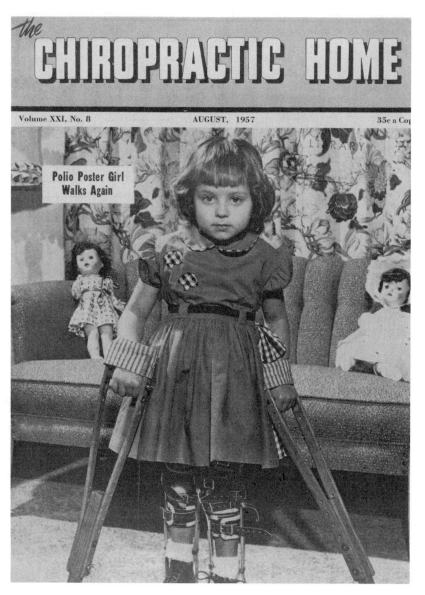

Winifred, the March of Dimes Poster Girl

INTRODUCTION

You may recall seeing photos in the mid-1950's of a girl named Winifred who was the March of Dimes poster girl. Her sweet sad face, huge crutches and cumbersome leg braces raised millions of dollars for the March of Dimes. Unfortunately, after two and a half years of medical therapy, she was given up as an incurable case. Her grandparents took her to see Dr. Lewis Robertson, a chiropractor. In fewer than six months, Winifred was walking without braces or crutches thanks to chiropractic care.

The irony of this story is that not one dollar of the millions she raised for the March of Dimes went to pay for the chiropractic care which allowed her to walk again.[1] Was it a mere coincidence, a spontaneous remission or simply a miracle? Read on.

On December 13, 1988 Dr. Greg Johnson of Austin, Texas and his wife were expecting their first children — six-week premature twins. Dr. Johnson is a chiropractor and told his wife's obstetrician they wanted a completely natural delivery without forceps or medication. Britney, the first twin, had a high forceps delivery, bruising her head and face and causing a blood clot on the head (cephalohematoma). The doctor also used twisting (torsional stress) on her neck during the delivery. Courtney, the second twin, was born without incident. The girls were 3 lb/6 oz. and 3 lb/8 oz. respectively. They were scheduled to be kept in the hospital neonatology department until they were at least five pounds in weight.

Within thirteen days of delivery Britney became very jaundiced. Her eyes were very yellow, and she had periods where her breathing stopped (apnea). The medical doctors were monitoring her blood and noticed she had hemolytic anemia, a condition where the red blood cells which carry oxygen were being destroyed faster than they could be replaced. This, coupled with the apnea, could have been fatal. The doctors wanted to perform a complete blood transfusion, which would give her normal blood but would not change the problem of the new blood cells being quickly destroyed.

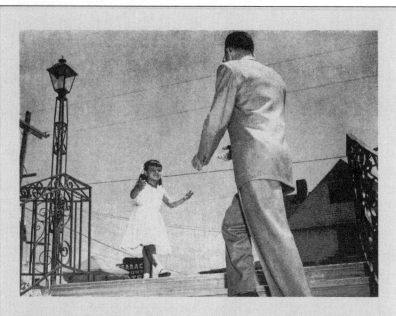

POSTER GIRL CURED

Instead, Dr. Johnson decided to try a spinal adjustment on his daughter. As the girls were identical twins, no one could say why Britney had this "rare disease" and Courtney did not. After checking her posture and noticing that her head tilted severely to the left, Dr. Johnson adjusted the highest bone in her neck (C1 vertebra) very gently. He did this four times the first day, three times the second day, and two times the third day. He said after the first day of adjusting that he watched the life begin to return to his daughter's eyes.

The medical doctors who wanted a court order to force a blood transfusion on Britney could not understand how she came around and had a full recovery without the aid of drugs or medical intervention. Dr. Johnson tried to explain how her nervous system had been damaged by the delivery, but they could not accept this explanation, any more than they could accept the idea that chiropractic care saved this child.[2] Was it a mere coincidence, a spontaneous remission or simply a miracle? Read on.

In September 1993, Dale Lineaweaver, owner and operator of Lineaweaver Racing, was test driving a motorcycle which he had designed and built. A second motorcycle was racing next to him. As they leaned over into the turn, the tailpipe of the second motorcycle, close to Dale's ear, suddenly emitted a loud blast. Dale's head reflexively snapped away to the side, causing his neck to whiplash. Within hours he developed a ringing in his ear which rose to over 40 decibels (about the sound of someone talking loudly directly in your ear).

His insurance company spent over $4,000 on diagnostic tests and therapy, none of which helped. After two months of frustration and being unable to work, he came to my office. After two adjustments to his neck the decibel level dropped in half. After one month of care the ringing was down to five decibels and dropped slowly over the next few months until it became almost inaudible. Ironically, his insurance coverage did not include chiropractic care.

All three of these true stories dramatically show how chiropractic methods worked when medical therapies failed. In two of the instances had insurance coverage been a barrier, the patients would not have gotten well or would have had to pay cash for care.

Purpose

My purpose in writing this book is to let you know that you are being robbed at this very instant! Something is being taken away from you that is your birthright as a normal functioning human being—your good health. Many doctors claim to cure you even though you refuse to change behaviors that can kill you prematurely. Ask no questions. Doubt not about the outcome. Simply take this pill, remove this organ, drink this tonic, and it will be as if you were never sick. But if something goes wrong, or if you are a little too good at killing yourself, no one could help you.

I am not implying that your health professional is intentionally out to rob you, but how often does your trusted medical doctor refer you to a chiropractor to regain your good health? Seldom, if ever and usually only for a nagging backache, sprain/

strain, crick-in-your-back type of problem. Well, I will challenge some concepts you may have about health because I want you to know where health really originates. I will even give you a hint: the answer is inside you right now. By the way, we are pretty darned good at fixing those backs!

In this book I focus and center on two things. First, I want you to have abundant health. Chiropractic care can help you get it and keep it. You will get step-by-step instruction on how to find a good chiropractor, what conditions you may have that chiropractic can help, and true stories of people whose lives have been saved or changed by good chiropractic care. In essence, I want you to see a chiropractor. Period. See one for an initial consultation and/or a spinal examination regardless of whether you think you need one or not.

If I were a dentist, I would ask you to see a dentist whether you think you need one or not. Indeed, the only reason you might not need to see a dentist is if you have no teeth. The same is true for this book — if you have no spine or nervous system, you may stop reading here!

When I looked in my local bookstore, I found a selection of books on back care. Most were written by medical doctors, orthopedic surgeons, massage therapists or yoga gurus. There were no current books written by chiropractors on the subject of back pain and health. Nor were there any books connecting these two crucial issues together. Most people are aware that chiropractors can help a bad back, but few know that we can help with asthma, high blood pressure, epilepsy, heart conditions, ulcers and many other "medical" problems.

After ten years of college to earn a Doctor of Chiropractic (D.C.) degree, I realized there was a need for more people to experience what I and my patients have come to understand — good health and a sound back go together. There are many "miracles" of good health which are gained from a healthy spine. For millions of people, there are no greater experts on the care and health of the spine than chiropractors. Chiropractic can help you regardless of your health, whether you are the fittest human being on the face of the earth, or someone who has been sick for many years. The only person that may not need to be adjusted is someone who has just been adjusted. I believe the only people we cannot help are those suffering from the disease known as "rigor mortis!"

Second, I must warn you, right now you are slowly losing your right to choose, not only your personal doctor, but also the kind of doctor you wish to consult. As you will see upon reading the book, chiropractic care gets results. In many cases it works better than alternative forms of treatment. Presently many insurance companies cover chiropractic care; however, many do not. Some insurers make you go through a medical doctor who acts as a gatekeeper to obtain a referral; this is true of Health Maintenance Organizations (HMOs). Many of the insurance companies that offer coverage put severe restrictions on the type of care available and the number of visits allowed.

Can you imagine what would happen if you needed heart surgery and the insurer only permitted one surgery limited to four hours and then two or three post-surgical visits? Or you could stay in the hospital four days and only have one set of lab tests—any additional care would not be covered.

This would be silly, unrealistic and dangerous. Unfortunately, some patients do forfeit necessary medical treatment due to finances. It's the same with chiropractic. If there has been a problem with your back for a long time, or you have had a bad accident causing trauma to your spine, it will take an extended period of time for the problem to improve.

One insurance company uses big ads which show a jellyfish floating in the water. The ad tells you that jellyfish have no spine and, according to many insurance companies, neither do you. This particular company states that it is proud to offer chiropractic care to its members, but you should always check the fine print to see the complete coverage.

You may want to ask your doctor of chiropractic which insurance companies have the best and fairest plans. Make sure the type of coverage you get avoids severe restrictions and limitations. Read the provisions carefully. It is up to you—the health consumer — to demand choices in the type of care you receive. I will speak more about this in the chapter on health insurance.

This book does not claim that chiropractic care works for every disease on the planet, nor does it bash the medical profession unfairly. Rather, I wish to disclose the benefits of chiropractic care and why it's the most powerful and least invasive way for the body to regain and maintain health naturally.

I want you to know why only a licensed doctor of chiropractic should adjust your spine, not an M.D. or physical therapist. I will show you ways you can attain and regain your health and save money by finding the right chiropractor for you and doing corrective back exercises. Finally, I want you to know exactly what a spinal subluxation is and how it can have devastating consequences to your health if you do not correct it.

This book is about health, what prevents you from the health you deserve, and how you can regain it. I hope you will be enlightened as well as entertained. In many instances I have included actual patient success stories, but in all cases I have changed the names or used initials to protect privacy. We all love to hear about people who have beaten the odds and gotten well, despite what others have advised. Any of these people could have been you, someone you love, or someone you know.

If parts of the chapters get too technical, skip them. Read only what interests you. I have included some of the more technical information only for reference, and even then limit it to the appendices. If you wish to learn about the benefits of chiropractic, how it helps, and also be entertained, then this book is for you. If you wish to learn some of the "hard science" behind chiropractic, this book is also for you. I hope you enjoy what you are about to read.

Background

This book comes out of years of frustration working in, and being a consumer of, professional health care in one capacity or another. Growing up in the early 1960s, our family did not consult a chiropractor. To us, chiropractors were heretics and witch doctors. Our attitudes were simply a result of negative propaganda by the American Medical Association.

My mother was a nurse for almost 40 years for Dr. Paul H. Ryan, a wonderful medical doctor in Richmond, California. Dr. Ryan was from the old school of medical training, as was my mother. At that time, physicians did not like chiropractors because they were uninformed of the benefits of chiropractic care. You may be aware that medicine and chiropractic are not the best of friends; indeed, until recently they have been bitter enemies. Due to recent developments in research showing that spinal adjustments can provide almost instant and lasting relief to those suffering from back pain, many medical doctors now grudgingly admit that there might be some therapeutic value to the science of chiropractic.

We chiropractors find this recent recognition rather amusing because we know people have been adjusting or manipulating the spine for thousands of years. Yet it was not until September 18, 1895 that the first "chiropractic adjustment" was given. Dr. D.D. Palmer, a magnetic healer, adjusted the back of his janitor, Harvey Lillard. Harvey had become deaf seventeen years earlier when he

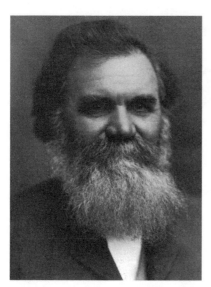 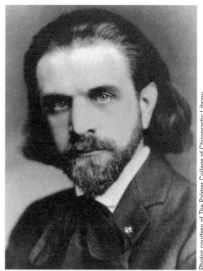

Photos courtesy of The Palmer College of Chiropractic Library

Left, D.D. Palmer, the founder of chiropractic (1905); right, B.J. Palmer, the developer of chiropractic (circa 1920's)

displaced a vertebra in his neck. Dr. Palmer grabbed the vertebra and in his words, "I racked it into position using the spinous process as a lever and soon the man could hear as before."[3] Almost immediately, part of Harvey's hearing came back. Over the next few days almost all of it returned.

Although this story may sound somewhat unbelievable, note this quote from J.F. Bourdillon, M.D.: "The start of chiropractic is said to date from a specific incident when Palmer manipulated the thoracic vertebrae of a Negro porter and by this means cured him of deafness which he had suffered for some years. On the face of it, this is a fantastic and totally unacceptable claim. As a result of personal experience, however, there is no doubt in my mind that somatic dysfunction in joints in the upper thoracic spine can affect the function of the inner ear, presumably by way of its sympathetic innervating."[4]

Chiropractic was never really intended for back pain. It is simply an accident (or nature's plan) that it helps sore muscles and ligaments and relieves back pain. Chiropractic is intended to help you live with optimum health, free from disease throughout your long, healthy life.

Another significant event over the last few years has also helped the chiropractic profession grow. The American Medical Association (of which not all M.D.s are members) was found guilty in court of carrying on a major campaign to destroy the chiropractic profession. Its members were neither allowed to refer patients to chiropractors, confer with chiropractors, nor associate professionally or personally with chiropractors. Believe it or not, they were even discouraged from dating or marrying chiropractors!

Yes, this lunacy was why a group of four chiropractors, Drs. Chester Wilk, Michael Pedigo, James Bryden, and Patricia Arthur sued the AMA for antitrust violations in 1976. They were represented by George McAndrews, Esq. They won their case in 1987 as Judge Susan Getzendanner handed down a 101-page opinion against the AMA. The AMA appealed the decision and lost in 1990 before the U.S. Court of Appeals. The case then went to the U.S. Supreme Court which refused to hear it. Eventually the

AMA had to admit guilt to its membership. It also had to tell the members they could now associate ethically and work with chiropractors on patient cases.

Lately, there is more hard scientific data to support chiropractors. Scientists and medical doctors, some trying to prove chiropractic a sham, have found that their research has actually proven just the opposite. Additionally, independent scientists, chiropractors and chiropractic colleges are conducting research to help prove what chiropractors have been maintaining for years — chiropractic works. It gets results and that's all that matters.

Today more and more M.D.s are referring patients to chiropractors, consulting with chiropractors, and even bringing chiropractors onto the staffs of major hospitals and medical centers around the country.

At one time I had planned to go to medical school. I took all the courses, the tests, and worked in surgery at John Muir Medical Center in Walnut Creek, California, one of the finest hospitals in the nation, in order to learn the practical aspects of the field. However, I became somewhat disillusioned of the life of a medical doctor. Many of the surgeons whom I liked and admired warned me of the many problems in medicine: the long hours, the futility of many cases, and the emergence of new insurance plans which take control away from doctors and place it in the hands of insurance executives. Most liked the practice of medicine but hated the business of medicine.

Many doctors were uncomfortable with the undesirable side effects of the powerful drugs they prescribed. After several years of testing on the general populace, some medications deemed safe for the patient showed themselves to be harmful. Some drugs even had side effects which were the same as the conditions they were supposed to treat! It was not uncommon to hear talk in the surgeons' lounge about a common medication or surgical procedure used for years which was suddenly taken off the market or banned by the authorities.

Years later I read *Confessions of a Medical Heretic* by Dr. Robert S. Mendelsohn.[5] This book gives incredible insight into thousands of mistakes in modern medicine, millions of dollars wasted each year on modern health care, and most importantly, many lives lost or permanently damaged by poor medical care. In order for you to better understand the adverse effects many drugs and surgeries have on your health, I strongly recommend that you pick up a copy of this book as soon as possible.

Another good book for some insights into the American medical establishment is *Medicine on Trial: The Appalling Story of Medical Ineptitude and the Arrogance That Overlooks It.*[6] Here, the authors go further into the medical system and show how self-limiting and self-sustaining it has become. They explore the risks of medicine and surgery, the unfortunate accidents which occur, the cover-ups and how the medical system has tried for years to eliminate any and all competition from non-physician providers—all at the expense of the public which it has sworn to protect. They say the biggest mistake that medical doctors make is to assume that they alone practice medicine. There are very strong financial motives for controlling or eliminating any other allied health system or provider. The authors caution that Americans are losing their ability to choose alternate systems of care which likely could be cheaper and more efficient.

When I decided to attend chiropractic school, I discovered that the philosophy of chiropractic was radically different from that of medicine. Chiropractic doctors believe that health comes from within the body rather than by adding drugs or cutting organs and body parts. The body can heal itself—what a concept! In the words of my friend Charles Ward, D.C., "God doesn't make any junk!"

Is it possible that those tonsils He gave you might come in handy some day? Why would you let someone routinely cut them out? When they inflame and get bigger, they are only doing their job, to remove dead white blood cells via the lymphatic system.

The differences between the chiropractic students and medical students I met were obvious—the chiropractic students seemed so happy to be there. There were many athletes and health enthusiasts; people had positive mental attitudes on campus. Even though the four-year curriculum that I saw for chiropractic students closely resembled that of medical school (to my dismay and horror), the chiropractic students seemed relatively relaxed and friendly.

By comparison, many of the medical school students I met were so stressed they could only give me a moment of their time. Of course, not all of them were this way, but it seemed to me that the majority of future chiropractors were happy and relaxed. They seemed to know that they were headed for a profession where they could help people regain their health and have a positive effect on lives, while earning a comfortable living and possibly making the world into a better place in which to live.

Finally, my own health had been in question. All my life I had been plagued by asthma, allergies, and frequent colds. Medication seemed to help the symptoms but did absolutely nothing to attack the underlying condition. I would ask the medical doctors what caused my health problems. No one had any answers; they just gave me more pills. True, when I began to take higher doses of vitamin C at the recommendation of Dr. Ryan, some of the symptoms disappeared, but never completely.

When I began to get my spine adjusted into the correct position by Dr. Daniel Murphy of Pleasanton, California, I noticed a radical improvement in my health. My asthma and allergies vanished completely, and they have not returned since.

I am pleased to hear my patients tell me that they are the only ones in their family not sick with a cold or flu that is going around. They start to understand that chiropractic is good for a lot more than painful backs. Chiropractors work on the nervous system of the body which controls everything, including the immune system. This is why they get fewer colds than other family members.

As you read this book, remember that not all people agree with me or this philosophy. In fact many people in the health care field prefer that chiropractors stay within their limited view of how they think we should practice. That's okay. Once again, more and more good, solid research is proving what doctors of chiropractic have known for years—this approach really works.

Chiropractic adjustments do a lot more than just alleviate back pain. If it were just a placebo, it would never have survived and flourished over the last 100 years to grow into the second largest health care delivery system in the world.

Most ignorance is either a lack of knowledge or a faulty understanding of certain concepts. The people who advise you against visiting a chiropractor may be reacting to some negative image they have been carrying with them. Perhaps they've had a negative experience with a doctor of chiropractic. In most cases the advice is intended to be in your best interest. It is not uncommon for someone to think that a particular chiropractor represents all chiropractors. Remember, it is possible that a particular chiropractor may have been unable to help, but it is not true that CHIROPRACTIC in general is ineffective. If you went to a lousy medical doctor, you wouldn't say MEDICINE in general is bad, would you?

I hope that after you read this book, you decide for yourself to try chiropractic. It is your life and your body. It's you who suffers from back pain and/or poor health, not other people giving advice. Chiropractic adds years to your life and life to your years!

W. Michael Gazdar, D.C., C.C.S.P.

Walnut Creek, California

November, 1996

What is Chiropractic — And What Will the Chiropractor Do for You?

The day you take responsibility for yourself is the day you start your climb to the top and back to health.

—David M. Amaral, D.C.

Definition

Chiropractic is the art and science of diagnosis and treatment of the spine, spinal disorders and disorders of the nervous system. It is a drugless and nonsurgical mode of care. A chiropractor is trained and licensed to practice the art of adjusting the spine ("manipulation therapy") and related joints of the body in order to restore proper motion to that joint, causing not only a restoration of function, but also leading to a decrease of local and distal nerve pressure. Local nerve pressure is a result of soft tissue swelling around the joint. Distal nerve pressure is a result of tethering or traction of the entire nerve at the affected joint or a result of abnormal spinal posture.

The translation of the previous paragraph is simply that vertebrae have misaligned due to some trauma or bad posture and caused swelling which affects a nerve and stops that nerve from carrying out its normal function. This may cause pain, degeneration, sickness, disease or even death. As a side note, many chiropractors do not like the terms "manipulation" or "therapy". These are medical terms and what we do is very distinct from medicine.

What You Need to Know

My goal in this chapter is to demystify exactly what chiropractors do, and what awaits you when you go to see a chiropractor for the first time. Remember, I cannot speak for the entire profession because every doctor of chiropractic is a little different in his or her approach. However, as an instructor at a chiropractic college, I can tell you what is taught as a customary approach to patient evaluation, diagnosis and management.

In order to acquaint yourself, you should carefully question the person who answers the phone in the doctor's office. Have a list of questions ready in advance. I suggest you ask the following questions:

1.   Will I be seen by a licensed doctor of chiropractic, who graduated from an accredited school of chiropractic?

2.   To what professional organizations does the doctor belong?

3.   How long has the doctor been in practice?

4.   Will I be seen initially by the senior doctor of the clinic or by one of the associates?

5.   Must I pay cash, or will they process my insurance forms? How much will the first visit cost?

6.   What hours does the doctor keep, and is the doctor available for emergencies?

7.   Does the doctor network with other health professionals and is he or she on any referral lists of other types of doctors?

8.   How long does the first appointment last?

9.   Anything else you feel is important to ask.

The following are things you should be prepared to answer.

1.   Have I ever been a chiropractic patient in that office before or anywhere else?

2.   What is the nature of my complaint?

3.   Is this an emergency?

4. Is this work-related? (Most on the job injuries are covered 100% for chiropractic by worker compensation.)

5. Is this the result of an auto accident? (Most personal injury cases are covered 100% for chiropractic by auto insurance.)

6. How quickly do I need to be seen by the doctor?

7. My phone number and address.

8. Who referred me to the doctor? (This is for the doctor's information only. Chiropractors are primary health care physicians. You do not need a medical referral to see one. However, your medical insurance might only cover you if you are referred by an M.D. This questionable practice hopefully is in the process of being repealed wherever it is in place.)

9. What type of insurance (if any) do I have, and will I need to bring in the forms?

The First Visit

The purpose of the first visit in most doctor's offices is to gather information. You will probably need to fill out standard health history forms. The doctor wants this information in order to get an overall sense of your health and your current chief complaint. Never leave off important information, such as personal or family history of asthma, strokes, heart disease, cancer, kidney problems, vascular diseases, arthritis, depression or other mental problems, or other major health conditions.

Next, the doctor or an assistant will interview you further to get a sense of your history and your reason for visiting the chiropractor. Even if you are there for a routine physical (which chiropractors are trained and licensed to perform) this information is very valuable. As with all doctors, your information will be kept in the strictest of confidence. It is said that after the history has been taken, 90% of the diagnosis can be made. This has certainly been true for me in my practice.

The doctor, or one of the associates will perform an examination to determine what is physically wrong and right with you. This practice varies greatly among chiropractors. When you go to a medical doctor's office for a routine physical, you usually know what to expect. The chiropractor will probably conduct almost the same exams as a general practitioner (family doctor), but with a heavier emphasis on the health and function of the spine and nervous system.

Unless requested, the chiropractor will probably not do a breast exam, pelvic exam, penile exam, rectal or prostate exam. In most states we are licensed to carry out these exams, but many chiropractors choose to leave these types of examinations to your medical doctor. However, if the chiropractor is the only doctor within many miles, he or she may have become the town's family physician and will perform all of the studies mentioned above.

The chiropractor will inspect the site of your chief complaint and probably other areas of your spine as well. He or she will probably percuss (tap) these areas and listen with a stethoscope to your heart, lungs, and abdomen. The ranges-of-motion of your spine and your extremities will be checked in order to evaluate how well or poorly your joints are functioning. Orthopedic tests will be done to check for joint damage, and neurological tests to evaluate your nervous system.

The doctor of chiropractic may elect to x-ray your spine or extremities in order to better evaluate their condition. The chiropractor may want to order lab tests, such as blood or urine analysis, to evaluate your body chemistry. Lastly, he or she may need to order special tests such as CAT scan or magnetic resonance imaging (MRI), or may want to consult with a medical doctor if there appears to be a medical problem.

Many M.D.s appreciate chiropractors referring a patient to them if a medical problem seems to exist. Some medical doctors refer patients back to a chiropractor when there are difficulties with a case that could be better managed chiropractically.

One former neurology instructor at Life Chiropractic College West and currently at Palmer Chiropractic College West, Dale Nansell, Ph.D., liked to tell of one incident which occurred a few years ago. A patient was in an auto accident in which his head struck the windshield and caused a slow bleed to occur inside the brain between the two hemispheres. The patient was examined and diagnosed in the emergency room immediately after the accident with a clean bill of health and was sent home.

He then went to the chiropractor for recurring headaches and neck pain. In a few days the chiropractor noticed the patient began to have sensation problems in his feet, his legs, and finally the trunk of his body. The chiropractor thought the patient might have a slow bleed in the brain and sent him to see a neurosurgeon immediately. Within a few hours the patient was on the operating room table having brain surgery which saved his life. The chiropractor later received a letter from the neurosurgeon praising him for his alertness in this patient's care.

In most cases the chiropractor will not adjust you the first day. He or she will need some time to go over your case and analyze exam findings and x-ray results in order to put it all together. A diagnosis is then made and a management plan is put together. However, if you are in a great deal of pain or have traveled a long distance, you may be adjusted that day. It is at the doctor's discretion.

You may be given an ice pack or some type of spinal or pelvic block and told to go home and apply ice. The ice will decrease the inflammation, and the block will help your spine start to move or change into the corrected position. Unless the inflammation has diminished (after an acute injury), it will be very difficult for the chiropractor to adjust the spine in that area.

If it is an acute injury, you should not use heat even though it might make you feel better. Heat causes the joint to swell more and produce more pain. Notice that in any professional sport when a player gets hurt, the trainer usually applies an ice pack to the injury site immediately.

Ruth is one of my favorite patients and the grandmother of my best friend while I was growing up. She used heat on her back and, although it made it feel better at the time, it would hurt worse later. Now she tells me that when she wakes up with back pain, she goes downstairs, gets her ice pack and carries it back upstairs to bed with her. A great patient is one who practices what her chiropractor preaches!

You should not use ice unless directed by your physician. There are some circumstances in which ice can be harmful: e.g., if you have a pacemaker, cancer, a weak heart, decreased sensitivity to cold, some vascular diseases, or have had frostbite. There is a section at the end of the book on the proper use of ice. *Do not use this book to self-diagnose and self-treat your condition.*

The Second Visit

At the second visit you will be given a report of findings. Now you will find out what the problem is, how long it is going to take to resolve it, how much it will cost, and whether or not it is going to hurt (it almost never does!). The doctor will tell you what he or she has found and what the best type of care is for you. If possible, you should have one or more of your family members present, especially someone you trust. You want them to support your coming to see the chiropractor in the future. If they have been educated about your condition, they are more likely to support the care you receive and encourage you to stay with the program of care that has been outlined for you.

Dr. Robert Mendelsohn, in *Confessions of a Medical Heretic,* says that what medicine has done is to try and make the patient passive and submissive. This is best accomplished by separating the patient from loved ones. He says the "New Doctor" will encourage the participation of the family in helping the patient regain health. Chiropractors are considered by many as family doctors and want participation of the patient's family.

At this second meeting the chiropractor should show you the results of his or her findings and then explain what all this means in terms of your health. The chiropractor will usually explain a little bit about how your body works and what went wrong in the first place.

The doctor will inform you about subluxations, what that means and the necessary course of action. He or she should explain that by restoring the vertebrae to their normal position joint integrity can be restored, pressure on the nerves eliminated, and your health regained. It's that simple. The power that made the body can heal the body, given the right environment for health.

The chiropractor will outline a program of care which is specific for your case. There is no way for me to tell how much care you will need as you are not my patient. I would never second guess another chiropractor's opinion unless I had examined you personally and reviewed your case history.

You should understand that there are usually three phases to care, but you may need less or more care depending on your specific condition.

Phase One: Pain Relief.   This is the first part of acute care. We try to relieve your symptoms by taking away the pain. The care here may be daily, or three to four times a week for a certain number of weeks, depending on your chiropractor's opinion of your case. Unfortunately, some patients quit care at the end of this phase and often return later in more pain because the underlying problem was never corrected.

Usually after a month or so the chiropractor will re-examine you and probably reduce the frequency of your care. As the tissues surrounding the vertebrae get more and more accustomed to being back in their proper position, they will hold that position for longer and longer periods of time. Thus, you will not need to be seen as frequently as you are holding your adjustment. Next comes the second phase of care.

Phase Two: Correction or Near-Correction of the Spine. This is the second part of acute care and also the subacute care phase. For the most part, you will probably have less pain. There will be times, however, when you have minor flare-ups as the ver-tebrae learn to live in their new corrected positions. Overall, you should see that you walk straighter, feel better and are more ener-getic, and possibly notice improvement of any other health problems you may have experienced. The care here may be once or twice per week for a somewhat longer period of time.

Phase Three: Stabilization, Maximum Health, and Prevention of Future Problems. This is the third phase of care, and many chiropractors believe this to be the most critical one. We have all heard the saying, "an ounce of prevention is worth a pound of cure," and this is very true. Here, the amount of care depends entirely on your condition. The frequency may be as much as once or twice a month, or as little as once or twice a year. Most people are somewhere between these extremes.

Unfortunately, many chiropractors, fearful of rejection by their patients, fail to recommend this important aspect of care. They don't want to be part of the "chiropractors make you come back to them for life" complaint. If you ask chiropractors how often they themselves and their families are checked and adjusted, most say at least once or twice per month — for LIFE!

If they want a long healthy, pain-free life for themselves and those they love, should it be any different for their patients who trust them? One of my colleagues, Dr. Ethan Feldman of Berkeley, California, says that when their critical care is completed, most of his patients prefer to come in once per month for maintenance "tune up" adjustments. In actuality, many patients come in for care not because they hurt, but because they don't want to hurt.

It is unfortunate that many people put a low priority on their health until it becomes critical. This is why so many emergency rooms are full. People wait until it becomes so bad that they need acute care. Then we have to return to the intensive care stage again.

Another concern of patients is money. Many do not see the need to spend anything on their health unless it is life-saving. Even then, insurance should take care of all of the bill. It is understandable in tough economic times to think this way, yet if the benefits outweigh the cost, isn't your health worth the price of a good dinner and movie?

Insurance may or may not cover all treatment aspects. If someone sees a chiropractor once a month (and pays between $25 and $50), it is not going to break them. The benefits they feel will generally be long term as their health improves. They save future doctor bills, time off from work due to illness, and have more time to play with their families. The care you get pays for itself. All this leads to reduced stress and a better state of mind. Dr. Darrell Lavin of Castro Valley, California, told me one of his patients came in after care and said with tears in his eyes, "This weekend I shot baskets with my son. I never thought I would ever do that again."

It also saves insurance companies and employers money as people get healthier and take fewer sick days. So, for around $400 per year you can have great health. This is the cheapest life insurance going. All of the care in the beginning may sound like a lot, but when you realize your back problems have been developing for a while, then you can understand why it takes some time to regain your health. If you went to an orthodontist, you would expect to be under care for awhile. It is the same with chiropractic.

Standard of care protocols for the entire chiropractic profession are being examined currently through what is called the "Mercy Conference Guidelines." These have set up approximately how many visits a patient might need if he or she has a strain of the muscles of the low back compared to a sprain of the ligaments of the low back or a disc lesion of the low back. Each successive problem is a more severe condition than the prior one and requires more visits. Some chiropractors are critical of this document because every patient is different and everyone responds to chiropractic at a personal pace.

The difficulty occurs when you consider the other factors which affect the patient's health. For example, if the patient smokes, is overweight, eats a diet rich in fats, exercises little, is older, and generally in poor health, you can expect much slower progress.

If the patient has repeatedly injured the same area and has not gotten corrective care, a worse prognosis can be expected. Even with the best care, there is likely to be some residual effects that may not be noticed until months or even years later.

Some of the toughest cases we have to deal with are post–surgical patients and patients who have been given steroidal injections in their joints. Dr. Dan Murphy, D.C., D.A.B.C.O. says a joint which has been injected with steroids may have avascular necrosis (death of tissue due to lack of oxygen) for up to a year.[7] If this happens, pain and altered joint function are likely to continue. Unfortunately, in many cases this procedure is recommended because the M.D. is running out of choices. He or she may feel something must be done, and this seems to be the best solution, short of surgery.

For example, D came to my clinic for care. He was 91 years young at the time and had severe neck pain. His medical doctor had given him twelve steroid injections in his lower neck, and now he was in really bad shape. There was so much stiff fibrotic tissue in his neck and shoulders that his head had shifted sideways to the right. He needed several months of care to regain his health.

What really infuriated his nephew who took care of him was that the government was happy to pay the medical doctor who had treated him for an unlimited number of visits. Yet they were only willing to pay for twelve chiropractic visits, when he needed many more than that. He told us that he had sent letters to President and Mrs. Clinton, his congressman and also the Department of Health and Human Services. He finally pushed them into paying the bill. Many times this is the amount of pressure it takes.

In considering a condition of inflammation around a joint, the common medical procedure would be to just remove the swelling with anti-inflammatory and diuretic medications. There are three problems with this course of action.

1. The swelling is there for a reason. The body is telling you not to move the joint—limit its use and let it heal. Unfortunately, the body sometimes overreacts and puts in too much fluid, and edema results. Some fluid needs to be released, but how much? Studies have shown that gentle range of motion exercises and chiropractic adjustments may help the joint pump out enough of the harmful edema, also known as inflammatory exudates.[8]

2. What is the actual cause of the swelling? It's one thing if the joint has had direct trauma, but if the problem originates somewhere else in the spine, then working on that swollen joint may help, but will never solve the problem fully.

3. The drugs which are used are very powerful. They cannot be expected to stop at just decreasing the swelling. They may start eating away at the normal healthy tissue and cause damage. This damaged tissue will also scar and cause more compression on the blood vessels, which will cause further scarring. It's a catch-22 situation. Scarring and avascular necrosis cause *more* scarring and avascular necrosis—it's an ongoing cycle.

Getting back to what you can expect on your second visit, the doctor may also be evaluating your emotional state concerning your health. Your state of mind can lengthen or shorten your case considerably. Kirby Landis, D.C. tells his patients that it used to be thought that a patient's mental state, either positive or negative, might affect his or her health. Now, there is no doubt about it. We know patients' mental states can help or hurt them, can make or break their case.

When a patient is stressed or feels the problem or condition is hopeless, he or she may have just destroyed a fast recovery. They could receive the best care from the best doctor, but they have effectively sabotaged any therapy and possibly made themselves worse. They are wasting the doctor's time and their own money.

On the other hand, if the patient tells themselves they will get better, overcome whatever the problem is, and have the best chiropractor working for their benefit, then they will surely get better. Chiropractors can instill in their patients a sense of confidence, backed up by the knowledge that the body is a self-healing organism. There is a force out there that only has to be released. Given the right nurturing environment, the patient will get well. There is a saying, "Whether you think you will get well or think you will stay sick, you are probably right."

Your case will determine the amount of care you need. Your doctor of chiropractic will recognize your individual needs and find a way to see you as often as necessary, but not more than necessary.

Once past the initial intensive period, you will, depending on your health "challenges," be seen only a few times per year. This may be every month, every other month, or every six months. I personally am checked every two weeks and adjusted about once or twice per month as needed. This keeps my asthma, allergies, and back pain away. If I am under increased stress or allow my diet to get sloppy, then I need to be adjusted more frequently. It's that simple.

Failure to Progress

If your condition has been present for a long time and you have hopes the doctor can "cure" your disease or organ problem, you must be willing to accept the fact that it may take time for your body to recover.

First of all, the body does all the curing. The chiropractor simply relieves the pressure on the nervous system so the nerves can begin resuming their normal function. This has the effect of healing the areas away from the affected nerves.

Second, if the nerve dysfunction has been there for quite some time, the damage may be rather extensive. If you are looking to the chiropractor for a quick cure, you may be disappointed. Usually the time it takes to cure the problem depends on how long the problem has been there. When the doctor gives you a program of care that has been tailored for you, he or she is expecting some degree of results in that time period.

Let's say you came in for low back pain and a chronic sinus problem. Suppose after three months of care with decreasing frequency of visits, your low back pain has cleared up, but you still have problems with the sinuses. It is possible the pressure on the nerves which go to your sinuses has been there so long there has been more damage than the doctor estimated. Your chiropractor may want to increase your visit frequency for a short period of time in order to get on top of the problem.

In other words, he or she may say, "I had hoped we would have your sinus problem handled by now, but it looks like one visit per week is not going to do it for us. What I want to do is check your spine daily for the next month and try to get the pressure off those nerves."

If it looks like you may resist this idea, having graduated from three visits per week to once a week, he or she might tell you, "We can keep doing what we're doing, but you will probably get discouraged. Instead of putting it off, let's experiment daily for one month and then we'll know if the damage to the nerves is permanent, or if there is some hope for recovery."

The doctor is not trying to take your money nor waste your time. He or she is honestly trying to tell you it is going to take a little extra effort to get the problem resolved. In all likelihood, this is because you have waited too long to get care, or you didn't realize that your body has been sending you messages that it's sick and needs attention.

It is important to listen to what your body is trying to tell you, rather than deaden the signal with painkillers and other potentially harmful drugs. It is one thing to take a mild analgesic to get through the first couple of days after surgery or trauma, but quite another to let yourself live on painkillers because you don't want to go to the doctor.

The Adjustment

The second visit is usually when you will get your first adjustment. As far as the actual physical adjustment goes, I have included a chapter on the various techniques and what they do. Since we put nothing into the body and take nothing out and only use our hands to heal, there are many many ways to do this. In the movie "Jacob's Ladder," Danny Aiello plays Louis, Jacob's chiropractor. Although his spinal adjustment looked a little rough and the sound effects of the vertebrae moving into place were a little louder than necessary, his technique appeared to be what is known as Diversified Technique. The movie even made Aiello out to be a hero, pulling Jacob out of traction in the hospital (he had hurt his back and said he couldn't move), taking him to his office and, with an adjustment, getting him to walk again. Although it may seem farfetched, we have had many patients literally crawl in to our office and walk out pain-free after an adjustment.

This is an example of one way chiropractors adjust. There are many different techniques. You may want to watch the doctor adjust some of his patients before he or she adjusts you. If this is a concern, simply ask. Most doctors would rather have you watch than have you not get the care you need because of your fear.

Remember that you may not feel instant relief after an adjustment. The muscles may be in spasm, holding your back in one tight position. The chiropractor will adjust the problem vertebrae into the corrected positions, but it may take several days for the muscles to relax completely and the pain to go away. If you have any questions regarding your care, never hesitate to ask your doctor.

Regardless of what you may have heard, adjusting the spine usually does not hurt. In fact, the more you are able to relax and let the doctor do what needs to be done, the better it will be. This is really the best part: relaxing and putting your problems in the hands of a professional. You are taking the first step towards a longer and healthier life. Congratulations!

Special Education Class

Many chiropractors offer a special education class to their patients. We sincerely want to educate patients in the care of their bodies. People are bombarded every day with advertisements saying you can do anything to your body and it will be okay. Take this pill or buy this drug and you will be fine. Sorry folks, it doesn't work that way.

The body is very forgiving, but you cannot do anything you want and get away with it forever. We educate people not only on the care of their bodies, but also on how the chiropractor sets them up to heal to their maximum efficiency.

In my class, I teach the five factors for good health:

1) Healthy Food

2) Regular Exercise

3) Proper Amounts of Sleep

4) Positive Mental Attitude

5) Sound Nervous System

I relate how each of these factors is important for health, how each can deteriorate and adversely affect your health, and finally how your chiropractor can help in each of these areas. I also show how the body is formed and how devastating a vertebral sub-luxation can be for you. My patients go away with a clear understanding about chiropractic and are usually eager to tell their friends and family members and bring them in to be checked.

If your chiropractor does not conduct presentations or classes, he or she may have prepared a chiropractic video for you to watch, or given you this book and told you to read it. In any case, it is the job of the doctor to educate the patient so you know what to do in order to regain and maintain health. If your chiropractor or you want to call me, my number is listed in the back of the book.

How Much Will It Cost?

The best person to tell you how much your care will cost is either the doctor or the office financial person. As an informed consumer, you should find out all charges up front. Getting stressed over a big bill may undo much of the good work which has been done on your back. One of the greatest leaders of our profession and one of my heroes is Sid E. Williams, D.C., founder of Life Chiropractic College in Georgia. Dr. Williams says, "We accept all patients regardless of symptoms or ability to pay." I have a great deal of respect for this man and his willingness to care for people, especially in this day and age when many doctors are making patients pay all costs up front, whether it is a hardship to them or not.

Most doctors, including myself, try to find a way to help the patient get what is needed. We generally charge the same fee for the same service regardless of whether or not the patient is paying cash, using health insurance, or is part of a personal injury case. Worker compensation cases usually have their own set fee schedules.

Many clinics have a sliding fee scale based on your income, and there is always the possibility of bartering for your care if you have a skill the chiropractor needs. In reality, this is how many people got the care they needed during the Great Depression. According to Dr. Kirby Landis, chiropractors are busiest during times of economic hardship because of the stress everyone is under and the adverse effect this has on their health.

Education and Licensing in the USA

Since the early days of the Palmers and the pioneers of chiropractic, the standards of chiropractic education in the United States have changed drastically. Many years ago you only had to subscribe to Dr. Palmer's model of health, pay the tuition, and spend six months in the Palmer School to be graduated a chiropractor of the "Palmer Method" (of course, you still had to pass the curriculum and Dr. Palmer's watchful eye).

Today, modern chiropractic college is four years (12 academic quarters) of full time studies, taking as many as 30 units of courses per quarter. At Life Chiropractic College West in San Lorenzo, California, classes begin at 7:30 am and go straight through until the late afternoon, Monday through Friday. The classes the students are taking are basically the same classes medical students are taking with a few exceptions.

Realize that the student must have already gone to a regular college and have passed all of the standard pre-med courses such as chemistry, physics, and biology in addition to a few general education courses. At the present time there is not a Bachelor of Science degree required for admission to most chiropractic colleges. However, this is being considered as requirements for admission become more and more strict. Some states require the

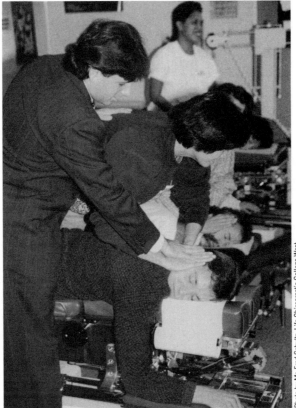

Technique instruction at Life Chiropractic College West in San Lorenzo, California. The four-year/12-quarter curriculum is the strongest in the history of the profession.

baccalaureate degree in addition to the D.C. degree for licensure in that state.

Suzanne Ray, M.S. is one of the most popular instructors at Life Chiropractic College West. She teaches a variety of science subjects including physiology and cardiovascular physiopathology. Like other great instructors, she takes difficult subjects and makes them easier by applying real life problems to abstract scientific principles.

Once she was on a long flight back East and happened to sit next to a cardiologist. Suzanne, who is no shrinking violet, likes to talk about her science classes and chiropractic. The cardiologist asked her what the chiropractic students learned about the cardiovascular system. After she explained it to him (it took about an hour), he stated that he was extremely impressed with the training.

Many higher education and medical professionals still do not realize the amount of material a chiropractic student must master in the four-year curriculum. The board exams, both written and oral, at the national and state levels are very difficult and take several days to complete.

Dr. Gerard W. Clum, President of Life Chiropractic College West, is one of the most intelligent and well-spoken leaders of our profession. He sits on many regulatory committees which supervise chiropractic education and practice in the United States. He has continued to push for high standards of chiropractic education as a necessity for the patient's sake. He has appeared before Congress to affirm the need for strong chiropractic education and a commitment of continued federal funding for chiropractic colleges. Patients deserve the best, and he is dedicated to turning out the highest skilled and most well trained chiropractors in the nation.

Postgraduate Work and Specialties

One of the best things about higher education and a professional career is that you can continue to learn and earn more advanced degrees throughout your life. In this regard chiropractic is like medicine and dentistry; there is no limit to the specialties and degrees you can acquire.

Many of the specialties are similar to those in medicine and require approximately the same amount of time to master with rigorous examinations. Fellowships are earned in chiropractic orthopedics, neurology, radiology, sports medicine/rehabilitation, and other subjects. There is no limit to the number of different techniques a doctor may study and attain proficiency. Some special techniques require full certification before they may be performed in the office.

Some procedures are limited to various states; each state has its own requirements to be licensed to practice chiropractic. In Oregon, doctors of chiropractic must pass a class in minor surgery, as they may be the only doctor within 500 square miles and may need to be able to suture bad lacerations and wounds.

Chiropractors in some states are allowed to prescribe minor pain-killers and anti-inflammatory medications. This upsets many traditional chiropractors who do not believe in taking drugs or medications. Indeed, it flies in the face of chiropractic, whose basic philosophy is that it is a drugless, surgery-free method of regaining your health.

Most of the advanced degrees such as the fellowships require several years of study and exams, and the pass rate is very low, due to the rigors of the course. Once the chiropractor has passed the exam, he or she may use the degree to advantage not only in patient care, but also if called to court as an expert witness or to work more closely with insurance companies in examining and evaluating patients.

In most states chiropractic care is covered 100% for personal injury cases and workers' compensation cases. Many insurance companies will request a second opinion if care is to continue for a long period of time or if the bill is abnormally high.

Now that you have a basic idea of a typical chiropractic visit, let's explore something we all possess but seldom think about: our spine.

2

What Does the Spine Do?

The doctor of the future will give no medicine, but will interest his patients in the care of the human frame, in diet, and in the cause and prevention of disease.

— *Thomas A. Edison*

These are the million dollar questions we need to answer: what does the spine do, why is it so important to good health, and why does it go bad or hurt so often?

The spine is one of the most important structures in the human body because it houses the most important system of the body, the central nervous system. The central nervous system consists of the brain and the spinal cord (the first section of the nerves which connect the brain to all other parts of the body). Diseases of the central nervous system are very debilitating and are often life threatening.

Hippocrates, the father of medicine, said, "Look well to the spine for the cause of disease." It follows that in order for a person to be healthy, he or she must have a sound nervous system.

Structural Problems and Trauma

There are two reasons the spine gives so many of us so much trouble. First, there is the basic structural problem. Humans are still in the process of making the transition of walking on two legs rather than four legs. I hope I won't offend any Creationists because I do believe in God! In reality, I feel chiropractors are doing His work of being healers through their hands. According to my late friend, motivational speaker Foster Hibbard, "God has never made a mistake and chiropractors are here for a reason."[9]

However you look at it, the spine has not developed sufficiently to do everything we demand of it and still hold up perfectly. There are weak areas: the design could be better; the bones and shock-absorber disc pads that lie between them could be stronger and more resilient; and the joints could wear out not quite as fast as they do. The blood supply to the discs could be more complete and last a lifetime instead of only the first two decades of life. Without blood, oxygen, and nutrients, the discs dry out and degenerate faster.

Second, our backs are subject to the trauma of everyday life, starting with the birthing process where the doctor, nurse or helper might pull a little too hard on the baby's unprotected head or neck. This is especially true if there is some sort of fetal distress, or if the mother hasn't dilated sufficiently and the situation becomes a medical emergency.

Growing up, there is the encouragement to walk before the baby is ready, even before it is ready to crawl. This can set up a condition in the low back where the lowest vertebra in the back (L5) has moved forward causing a type of sway-back (anterospondylolisthesis), which can cause low back pain for the rest of life. Of course, as the baby tries to walk, he or she falls down—again and again. If the fall is hard enough, it can knock vertebrae out of place (normal alignment or normal position) and cause swelling which compresses or pinches the nerves.

Another problem with walking before crawling is that important neurological connections are made as a baby crawls. According to Jim Hawkins, M.S., at Life Chiropractic College West, infants who are not allowed to crawl may carry these neurological deficits for life. So, let'em crawl!

Later there are all the fun childhood games which continue on into the teens and adulthood, such as dog pile (dogs don't even do this!), football, rugby, tumbling and gymnastics, to name a few. I cringe whenever I see a game of high school football and a player is hit from behind in the spine. Don't get me wrong, I love football. I used to play all the time as a kid, but now I know how lucky I was to escape any serious damage.

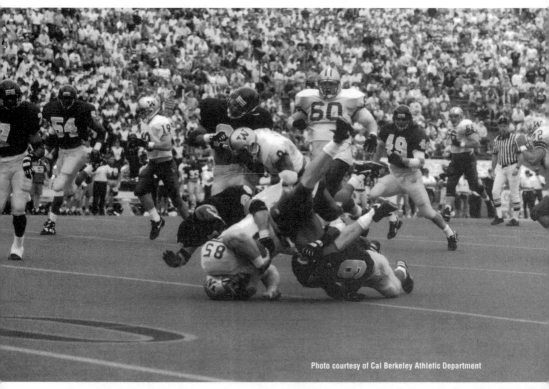

Photo courtesy of Cal Berkeley Athletic Department

College football is only one step away from the pros. Many teams keep a chiropractor on call for these types of injuries.

Problems occur because the spine does not completely become bone (a process called ossification) until a person is in their mid-twenties. Picture your child running with the football. If he is an average 14-to 17-year-old running back, he weighs 100-150 lbs. Now, here come two or three linebackers, each weighing about 150-220 lbs, aiming to spear your son (or daughter) and bring him down. There is not much protection for the delicate nerves of the spine.

Indeed, it is a wonder that more kids are not paralyzed by some of these activities. I'm not saying you should forbid your child from playing, but there needs to be some kind of extra support and protection on the spines of the players. That goes for the pros as well!

It is true that high school and college football has sent many good players to chiropractic college because chiropractic was the only thing which helped them after a traumatic hit. This has happened to more than one of my colleagues. One was injured while playing football. His spine was damaged and he spent six months in a body cast. The M.D.s couldn't do anything for him, so his parents took him to a chiropractor. The chiropractor restored full motion to his spine, and thereby cured his asthma, fixed his allergies, and also got him motivated to pursue the rewarding career of a chiropractor. He has helped thousands to regain their health and is now a leader in our profession.

When it comes to football, one wrong hit to the back, occurring in the blink of an eye, would not only end your football career, it could end or severely damage your life as well. It is no wonder there is a severe penalty for what they call clipping (hitting a player in the back). However, in the heat of the game there is bound to be one, if not several blows to the back.

Anatomy of Your Body

When you examine the anatomy of the body, it is really quite remarkable. The brain is on top controlling everything. The way it controls the rest of the body is through a network of wires called the nervous system. The nervous system consists of two segments:

1.   The central nervous system, which is the brain and the spinal cord (also known as upper motor neurons).

2.   The peripheral nervous system which consists of the nerves exiting the spine (also known as lower motor neurons). The nerves also are part of each spinal segment. The peripheral nervous system is composed of three parts: (a) sensory nerves which relay sensation back from the body into the spine; (b) motor nerves which relay messages out to the body to perform various motor functions such as movement of the body; and (c) autonomic nerves which control all of the unconscious functioning of the body such as glandular secretions, digestion, blood delivery, and heart rate. These nerves also control the visceral functions of the body, meaning all of the

internal organs. The functions are activated mainly by areas located in the spinal cord, brain stem and hypothalamus.

The autonomic nervous system is further divided into two parts: (a) The parasympathetic nervous system which is the system at work mainly while we are at rest. The nerves for this system rise predominantly from the cranial nerves in the brain and the sacral nerves at the base of the spine. (b) The sympathetic nervous system is the system which controls all of our "fight or flight" mechanisms. The sympathetic system also controls the amount of blood delivered to every organ in our body. There will be more on this aspect later. The sympathetic system generally exits the spinal cord between the base of the neck (T1) and just above the tops of the hips (L2). There is overlap as the nerves move up the neck and down the low back.

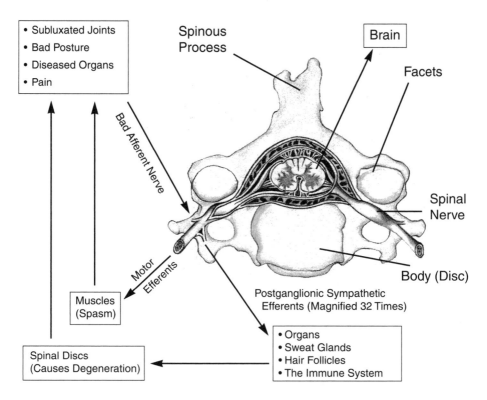

Simplified cross-section of the nerve loop in the spine, looking from above.

Just as the wires in your house must be protected, so must the brain and nervous system be protected. The skull protects the brain, while the bony spine protects the spinal cord. The spine is made up of 24 moveable bones called vertebrae, with small shock absorber disc pads between each bone. The spine acts as a conduit around the wires of the body. The rest of the nerves are protected by the soft tissue surrounding them, as well as the deeper structures of the body such as other bones, tendon sheaths, muscles and organs.

Nerve Dysfunction

The brain and nervous system are very delicate; it takes very little pressure to damage them. A vertebra may shift out of position and cause swelling and pressure on the nerves which exit the spine at that point. The swelling may produce only a few millimeters of pressure, but enough so that all or part of the nerve transmission is altered. This is what chiropractors refer to as a "subluxation."

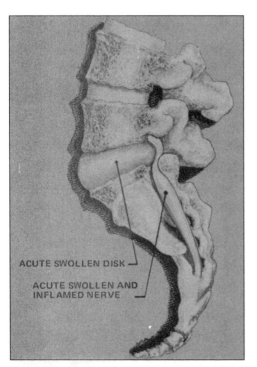
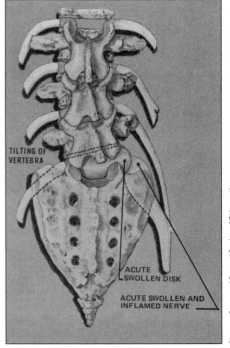

ACUTE SWOLLEN DISK

ACUTE SWOLLEN AND INFLAMED NERVE

TILTING OF VERTEBRA

ACUTE SWOLLEN DISK

ACUTE SWOLLEN AND INFLAMED NERVE

Diagrams Courtesy of Gonsead Seminar of Chiropractic

Side and back view of the lumbars, sacrum and coccyx. Here the L5 disc is swollen, showing compression on the L5 nerve. The L5 vertebrae is "subluxated".

Another way the nerves may be "pinched" is when a disc starts to degenerate. The disc may push backwards into the nerves in the spinal canal. This is known as a protruding or prolapsed disc. Along with the bad disc may come a degeneration or enlargement of the facet joints (small flat plane surface on the vertebrae which makes up part of the vertebral joint). As the nerve begins to exit the side of the spine at that level, it may also become pinched. Another problem can occur if there is not enough room in the center of the spinal canal (central canal stenosis).

All of these conditions can be helped with good chiropractic care. Each case is handled differently by your doctor of chiropractic. The causes of these conditions and how they may be remedied will be discussed in greater detail later in the book.

The one common "treatment" the chiropractor performs with each of these conditions is to take the pressure off the nerves by breaking the reflex that is causing muscles to tighten and sensory beds to react dysfunctionally. Another thing each of these conditions has in common is that the longer you delay care, the greater the damage done to the nerves and joints and the more difficult it will be to correct the problem.

During times of good health, the brain and spinal cord communicates 100% of the time with 100% of the body. When there is sickness and disease, something happens to that vital communication. It stops or the correct messages are sent, but at the wrong time or to the wrong place. Communication is two-way; the brain both sends and receives. It is no wonder things can go wrong; everything is so very complicated!

The nervous system is sometimes portrayed as an old-fashioned telephone switchboard. Picture several rows of wires with plugs on the end and then several rows of holes on top. When a call comes in, it is up to the operator to plug the right wire into the right hole to make the proper connection. Now multiply this by several million wires and holes that all have to be coordinated at once. The brain is the computer which does this every second you are alive.

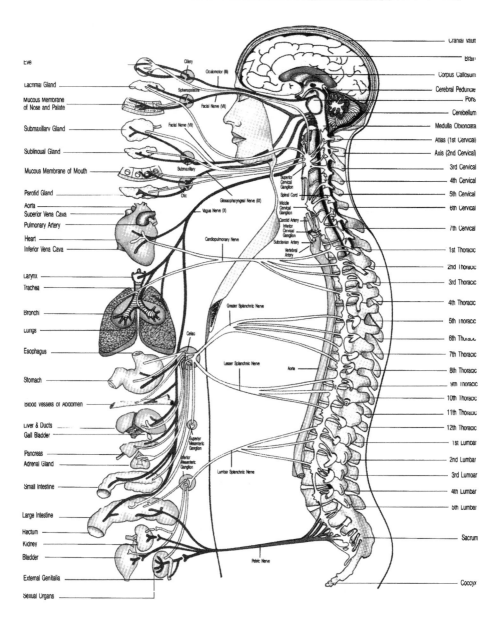

Diagram courtesy of The Parker Foundation

Autonomic Nervous System

Before we go further, we must establish one principle: the body moves naturally toward health. It is always trying to make itself healthy. It does not want to be sick or diseased. In fact, many of the things we call diseases, such as fevers and allergies, are simply the body's normal healthy reaction to fighting "dis-ease" (a chiropractic term). For example, a fever tries to kill something foreign in the body such as a virus or bacteria.

Pain is merely a warning sign of something wrong beneath the surface, and the spine is an excellent transmitter of pain. Very often when something goes wrong in the body, there is pain relayed somewhere. Each level of the spine sends nerves to different areas in the body in an orderly way. This informs us which organ is diseased or distressed.

One level of the spine corresponds to the function of the heart; another level might send nerves to control bladder functions. As an example, when someone has an attack of gallbladder stones, pain is often felt in the right lower tip of the shoulder blade. Heart attacks will often cause pain in the area between the shoulder blades.

A chiropractor is skilled in knowing whether the pain you feel in your back is the result of a spinal problem or a cry for help from some other part of the body. To illustrate this point, whenever I see a male patient over the age of 50 who comes in for low back pain, I routinely ask when he last had a prostate exam. It is known that prostate cancer or even inflammation of the prostate (prostatitis) causes low back pain. It is also known that prostate cancer is one of the biggest killers of men over the age of 50.

It is not that we are overly cautious, yet it is the doctor's job to be sure. This is why the history of the patient is so important. If a patient wakes up with pain one day and has problems with urination and there is no history of trauma, then one might consider prostate trouble. If he has fallen off a ladder onto his back, then chances are pretty darn good it's simply his back. Get the picture?

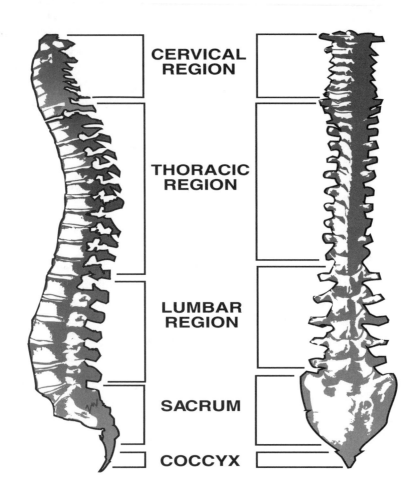

CERVICAL
REGION

THORACIC
REGION

LUMBAR
REGION

SACRUM

COCCYX

The side and front view of the spine.

Structure and Function

Another function of the spine is to keep us walking upright. It supports us and allows us to move about freely. It also provides an anchor for our muscles to attach themselves. We use it as a lever to lift heavy objects, and it functions to support our shoulders, arms, hips and legs. Obviously this is critical for us to be mobile, normally functioning human beings. Anyone who has had permanent back damage knows the limitations he or she now experiences, even though modern science has provided these special patients many options for getting around. No one likes to be dependent on another person for anything; the more they can take care of themselves, the better.

When you examine the skeletal system, you observe that the joints are at the best angles for making motion possible. The body is symmetric and functional. Each part has a function which interrelates and communicates with the rest of the body for complex movement and action. All of this structure, strength and mobility is dependent on the full coordination and cooperation of the brain, nerves, skeletal system, glands, and organs. The brain controls it all—the nerves housed in the spine relay messages to and from the brain and the rest of the body. It is complicated and must remain in balance at all times. Let's look closer at different parts of the back. Dysfunction in each area will be discussed in a later chapter.

The Neck (Cervicals)

The neck is known as the cervical region and is composed of seven vertebrae. It is the area of the spine closest to the brain. If there is damage to the neck, it can cause problems all the way down the spine, as well as to many different areas of the body. The cervical vertebrae are the smallest of the spine, yet they have the unique feature of carrying two large arteries up to the brain through their transverse processes (bony branches on each side of the vertebrae used for anchoring ligaments, tendons and other support structures). The arteries are called the vertebral arteries. The neck is divided into three regions:

1. **Upper cervical (occiput [C0], atlas [C1], and axis [C2]) region.** The brain stem protrudes at different times of the day down through these vertebrae. This region of the neck is the closest to the brain itself. Vertebrae out of place (subluxations) in this area usually cause pain and can be associated with many problems affecting the patient's overall health. This is the region which controls the majority of the blood supply to the head and influences the blood pressure and

heart rate via the vagus nerve. In fact, all of the nerves of the head (cranial nerves) are affected by this area.

2.   **Mid-cervical (C3, 4, 5) region.** This is the region of the neck which is responsible for supporting the normal curve of the neck. It is under a great deal of pressure due to the weight of the head and the stress of movement. According to Ruth Jackson, M.D., C5 is the major stress vertebra in the cervical spine. This is the vertebra which may be most adversely affected by direct trauma, such as a whiplash type of injury.[10]

3.   **Lower cervical (C6, 7 and T1) region.**   This is the base of the neck. It is the area where the shoulder joins the neck; nerves leading into the arms exit the spine (Nerves C5-T1). Any activity which causes the head to be thrust forward for extended periods of time, such as driving, sitting at a desk, working on a computer, or cutting hair can cause pain here and into the trapezius muscles, as well as pain, numbness, or tingling in the arms or hands.

The Mid-Back (Thoracics)

The mid-back is known as the thoracic region. It extends from approximately the level of the shoulders to the region known as the small of the back. There are 12 thoracic vertebrae and a disc between each of them. These vertebrae are unique in that each one holds a rib on each side. The top ten ribs on each side move downward and around the body and join in the front. As they join together they form what is known as the sternum.

The sternum extends down from the neck to just above the stomach. The rib cage houses and protects vital organs, such as the heart, lungs, spleen, part of the liver and the great blood vessels of the chest. At the bottom front of the rib cage is the diaphragm, which makes us happy by causing air to move in and out of our lungs (or annoys us by going into spasms and causing hiccups).

The two lowest thoracic vertebrae (T11 and T12) have small ribs attached to each side. These ribs (two on each side) do not attach in the front. They partially protect the kidneys on each side, but are rather delicate and may fracture if punched or hit.

From the side, the curve of the thoracic vertebrae is opposite that of the neck and low back. It thrusts outward, away from the body, like the hump on the back of the grey whale (or Quasimodo the hunchback if you are into horror movies!). More room is needed for the organs in this region, and by curving out, more space is created. This allows the lungs to expand to a greater volume, deliver larger amounts of oxygen to the tissues and exhale more carbon dioxide waste from the tissues.

The curve is called a kyphotic primary curve because we have it at birth and it changes little throughout our lives. In the womb we are in the fetal position, with our head bent forward and our knees drawn up to our chest. It is interesting that many people return to this position as they go into deep sleep.

The Low Back (The Lumbars)

The low back is known as the lumbar region. This region of the back is most important for holding the body upright. It is this part of the back which carries the most strain and consequently has the most structural problems due to physical stress. There are usually five lumbar vertebrae, each with a disc between them. However, some people have shorter backs, with only four lumbar vertebrae, and some people have longer backs with six lumbar vertebrae. Anything other than five is known as an "anomaly" and is discussed in the appendix entitled "Anomalies of the Spine".

The lumbar region is similar to the neck (cervical) region in that both have the same type of defined secondary curve, formed as the infant starts to stand up on two legs. Yet that is where the similarity ends. The vertebrae of the low back are the biggest of the spine. They have to support the entire trunk and head and are structured for support and free motion, including bending, rotating and flexing.

The spinal cord itself (the contained nerves) ends at about L1 or L2 in a structure known as the conus medularis and becomes the filum terminale. The nerves descending beyond this are in individual strands and are known as the cauda equina which means "horse's tail" (that is what it looks like!). The nerves move down the spinal canal and out the sides of the low back into each leg. This is similar to the nerves going into the arms from the base of the neck. Nerves also continue out to the organs in the pelvic region.

The Pelvic Region

The pelvis is comprised of two hip bones, each of which is a combination of three bones (the ilium, the ischium and the pubis), and the triangular-shaped bone called the sacrum. The sacrum is actually five bones that once were like vertebrae at the end of the spine but have all fused together to form one bone. The sacrum is the stabilizing base of the spine and fits together with the hips in a way that offers a great deal of stability and mobility.

The joints of the pelvis are the sacroiliacs in the back (where the sacrum and ilium join on each side) and the pubic symphysis in

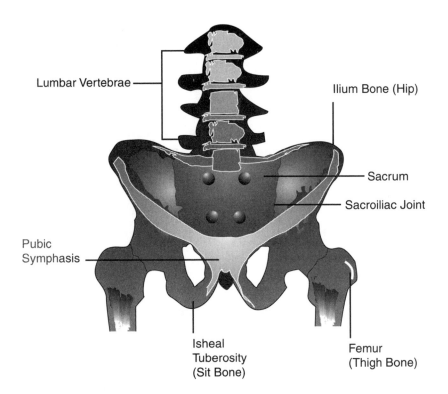

The front view of the pelvis.

the front (where the lower part of the hip bones, called the pubis, come together). The pelvis is attached to the lumbars by the lumbosacral joint and to each leg by the hip socket (acetabulum).

Problems which may occur include the sacrum rotating out of its normal position, causing one of the hips to rotate forward and up or backwards and down. This might affect either the sacroiliac or the lumbosacral areas. This is very common and can be corrected quickly with an adjustment by a chiropractor.

Trauma to the leg, hip, knee, or foot can cause the femur bone of the thigh to jam or twist into the hip socket. This is also addressed by chiropractic adjustments.

Another problem may be that the two pubic bones may not come together properly due to trauma or deformity. Bill Ruch, D.C., a chiropractor in Oakland, California and a former instructor at Life Chiropractic College West, has perfected an adjustment of the pubic arch which has helped even stubborn cases of pelvic pain. He tells of one instance where a woman, who had been married for five years, came to him suffering from pelvic pain. She had been in an auto accident soon after her marriage and, because of her pain, had been unable to have sexual intercourse since the accident. With one adjustment to her pelvis, Dr. Ruch alleviated the pain entirely, and she has been fine ever since. He promptly received a dozen roses from her grateful husband!

At the end of the sacrum are four to five even tinier bones fused together called the coccyx. Some say (sorry, Creationists!) that this is the remnant of the tail of our ancestors. The coccyx doesn't do much except act as an anchor to some important ligaments and add stability to the spine.

Often you don't feel or even think about the coccyx. It just hangs out and tries to stay out of trouble, unless you happen to fall down hard on your rear end. Then, if the coccyx has been jammed forward, it begins to hurt. Now suddenly you are reminded you have one! You may experience constipation or pain as you move your bowels, or you may have rectal pain if you sit for an extended period of time. Suzanne Ray, M.S. at Life Chiropractic College West, when teaching about this would say, "Rectum? Rectum? Why, it darn near killed 'um!"

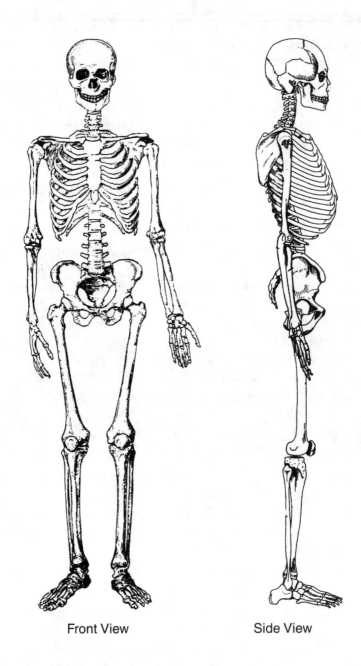

Front View   Side View

The human skeleton. All joints are at the proper angle for movement, support and stability.

Posture: The Normal Curves of the Spine

What are the normal curves of the spine? Like many people you may think your spine is straight, like a column which holds up the roof of a house's porch. This is not the case! As you look at the diagram, notice how the spine (when viewed from the front) looks almost straight. Don't worry, I didn't lie. From the front, the ideal spine would be straight, sitting on the two level hip bones making up the pelvis, with a straight spine and head on top. Everything is balanced and relaxed. The muscles are not overworking to correct a bad posture, and the small ligaments which join bone to bone are not being stretched into abnormal positions like a pretzel (unless you are a student of yoga!). This is what many chiropractors are trying to achieve.

Now look at the side view of the ideal spine. It's no longer straight! There are three main curves, one facing forward and two facing backwards. These curves also have an ideal position and degree of curvature. For each of the three curves, you should have between 30 and 60 degrees of curvature.

How these curves are formed is interesting. As most parents or older sisters and brothers can tell you, when a baby is born there is only one curve: the fetal position or primary curve. This is the curve which is in the middle of your back. It is maintained by powerful back muscles and the rib cage. At the age of a few weeks or months the baby begins to lift his or her head, and thus the neck curve begins to form. After the baby has started to crawl, he or she begins to stand and walk upright, and thus the curve of the low back is formed. The curves of the neck and low back are called secondary curves because they are formed second, after the curve in the middle of the back.

Most people, including chiropractors, do not have perfectly formed spines. In fact, many chiropractors have very bad backs. When nothing else worked, they were so impressed with the care and relief they experienced at the hands of other chiropractors that they became one themselves. So, for most of us who have less than the ideal back, what can be done to help us?

According to the posture-oriented technique known as Biophysics, developed by a chiropractor named Don Harrison, the best way to stop symptoms and increase the overall health of the patient is to identify the areas in the spine that are less than ideal (according to the previously explained postural model) and make them ideal. From an engineering perspective (he holds advanced degrees in mathematics), this is sound logic. Those of us who practice his technique do get amazing results as posture returns to normal.

It is usually easy for patients who have not been adjusted for some time to know when they need to be checked. They may notice that a shoulder is lower on one side. Their head may be tilted as they shave or put on makeup, or perhaps they walk with a limp because one leg is shorter than the other and their pelvis is being torqued.

One of my patients said that in every school picture as a child, and later as an adult, her head tilted off to the right. After two adjustments it straightened and only occasionally slips back into its old position.

You should be aware that there are many subdisciplines in chiropractic. In other words, we don't all do the same thing or treat patients the same way. Chapter 6 explains the different techniques and is important for you to read, enabling you to choose the type of technique which may be most suitable for you.

One of the most common ailments of the spine is postural scoliosis. Although it is a potential source of trouble, it may never hurt and consequently often goes unnoticed for many years. This illustrates that many things may be causing you spinal problems, yet may never "hurt" in the classic sense.

Scoliosis

When someone tells a person they or their children have scoliosis, it is often like yelling "shark" on a crowded beach. You get that gut-level reaction that churns your stomach. Or, if you are totally and blissfully unaware of what scoliosis is, you might say, "what?"

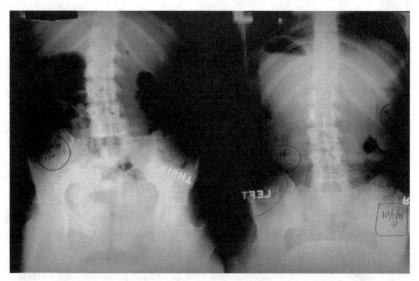

Before and after treatment of a scoliosis patient. This 35-year-old female presented with a 19° left scoliosis on 5/10/94. After being adjusted 2-3times/week, for five months, her curve had decreased to 9°. (10/1/94)

Scoliosis in its simplest form means abnormal curvature of the spine. Going back to our model, I said that the spine should be straight when looked at from the front. With a scoliosis patient you would see a definite curve that does not belong there. Instead of being straight from the front and back, the spine would appear curved. This curve may assume many forms. It may simply move to the side, or it might compensate in an "S" shape. This "S" shape may appear in one area of the spine such as the lumbars or the thoracics, or it may spread out over the entire back. As you might guess, gentle stretching, adjusting and tractioning is how to treat scoliosis patients.

From the side view, the spine may be deformed in a forward or backward direction. There are no set rules on how it may form or deform. Often we see a normal low back and the thoracics and neck straight and jutted forward. However, there are rules of classification. As an aside, if you suspect you may have some abnormal curvature of the spine, check your kids and other members of your family. It is a known truth that back problems are hereditary, just like other problems such as cancer, heart disease, and high blood pressure.

Here are two ways to check your children for scoliosis.

1.   Stand them up in front of you, preferably wearing their underwear or bathing suit and facing away. Look at the back for differences in hip or shoulder height, neck or head tilt, or obvious curves in their spines.

2.   Lie them face down on a bed with their shoes on. Straighten them out and look for a difference in leg length; one may be shorter than the other.

If any of these conditions exist, have them checked at once by a good chiropractor.

There are two major forms of scoliosis: functional and structural. Functional scoliosis is a curvature of the spine which becomes straight when the patient stands and then flexes forward at the waist. This means the vertebrae are moving in place with the back. This kind of scoliosis has a better prognosis than a structural scoliosis.

Structural scoliosis is a curvature which does not change when the patient bends at the waist. The vertebrae are essentially "stuck" in place. Very often as the patient bends at the waist, you will see a hump in the back. You may see one shoulder or shoulder blade higher than the other. For women, one breast may appear larger than the other.

Scoliosis has a variety of forms and causes, many of which will not be detailed here as there are many fine books on the subject. Here we will concentrate on some of the specifics and deal with chiropractic care, if applicable. You should recognize that scoliosis is a disease which may often continue its progression over time until the body becomes totally deformed, and the organs of the chest and stomach are compressed and unable to perform their normal function. As far back as 1958, German researchers found that 90 out of 100 instances of **stomach ulcers** were attributed to scoliosis in the mid-back (T6-T9). The researchers attributed this to pathological changes to the nerves, ligaments and discs of the spinal region.[11]

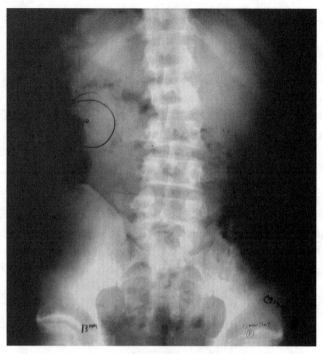

17° right scoliosis caused by a 13mm short right leg.
Notice how the spine curves toward the short leg.

When you consider that 90% of peptic ulcer patients had scoliosis, it is amazing how medical doctors treat ulcers in this country. Rather than giving drugs to treat the symptoms, why aren't we referring patients to chiropractors to get to the cause of the problem?

Scoliosis is generally not something out of which your child will grow. It may be self-limiting or it could get worse with time. There is an interesting observation known as the Hueter-Volkmann principle which shows that the spine will grow longer on the side that is less compressed and grow less on the side that is more compressed. In a growing patient, this could result in permanent wedge-shaped vertebrae.

This means that when the vertebrae are curved (concave) to the left, the majority of bone growth will be on the right. Thus, the curve to the left will continue to grow worse to the left!

Eventually, and at a different level, the spine will usually come back to the right as a compensation. This forms the "S" shape that we have been discussing.

This is where chiropractors can help. We will do everything in the opposite direction of the scoliotic curve. We will stretch the patient, adjust the vertebrae back into the correct position, use postural adjusting for correction (Certified Chiropractic Biophysics practitioners), and give the patient exercises which will help stretch out the back. Some of these exercises are detailed in the exercise chapter of this book.

The goal is to take the pressure off the compressed areas of the spine so that it will grow more normally. With the pressure off the concave side, there will be more growth on that side. With more pressure on the convex side, there will be less growth on that side. The patient should grow straighter. If your children are still growing, we can correct scoliosis more easily than if they have stopped growing. This is why they should be checked as early as possible.

In an advanced case the patient may have to be sent to an orthopedist for a consultation. In cases of severe scoliosis an orthopedist may want to use a brace between chiropractic adjustments. If the scoliosis is extreme or life threatening, surgery may be called for.

When evaluating someone for scoliosis, it is important to look at their posture both from the front and the side. If there appear to be likely scoliotic changes in the spine, an x-ray should be taken. In my office we do not take x-rays of children except in cases of trauma or suspected scoliosis. I use these films not only to measure the degree of scoliosis but also to help predict how much more growth a patient will have. There are specific laws concerning the care of patients with scoliosis, including guidelines for referral to orthopedists and other caregivers.

One frequent cause of scoliosis is one leg being shorter than the other. We measure patient leg length by tape measure. In addition, we examine the film of the pelvis from the front. The patient is standing on a level floor and is not leaning to either side as the film is being taken. The patient stands during the x-ray in order to evaluate the spine when bearing weight. In this way we can tell if one top of the leg (femur head) is higher than the other. We also look at the height of the hips relative to each other. Usually if there is no more than 6 mm (1/4 of an inch) difference, then a simple adjustment to bring the low hip up and the high hip down will be effective. Alternatively, if the patient has more than a 6 mm discrepancy, then a heel lift or a sole lift is often needed to make up the difference.

Dr. Dan Murphy has advanced degrees in chiropractic orthopedics and treats many scoliotic patients. He described one interesting case where a mother who had scoliosis brought in her 16-year-old daughter for care. At the time the daughter had a curve in her back of 24 degrees, which is fairly serious. It had been progressing for many years. After a few months of care, Dr. Murphy had stopped the progression and even straightened it a few degrees.

The mother then brought in her 12-year-old daughter who had a scoliosis of 11 degrees, and he treated the child the same way. The mother was delighted with his success. Her only regret was that she hadn't brought her children in to see him earlier. It was interesting that they each had one leg shorter than the other. This seemed to be what was causing their backs to be off balance.

It is worthwhile noting that there is not always a direct correlation between the degree of scoliosis and the length difference of the legs. One of my favorite patients is S. He broke his leg in an auto accident and had treatment requiring pins and surgery. He was 24 years old at the time of the surgery and most of the bone growth was completed. He came to see me for very mild low back pain ten years later when he was 34; he knew he had some sort of problem.

We took x-rays of his low back and discovered that his right leg was 29 mm shorter than his left leg! He had a 14 degree scoliosis with the apex to the right. He is very athletic but had never been given a heel lift to balance out his pelvis and spine. Now that S wears his heel lift, his back is much straighter and more balanced.

Then there is the case of B and his sister T. Both came to see me because they had been in an auto accident and had been whiplashed. They had severe neck pain and headaches. We noticed on the films that they each had one leg shorter than the other. B, who was 18, had a right short leg of 10 mm and a right apex scoliosis of 12 degrees in the lumbar area. T, who was 15 at the time, had a 15 mm short left leg and a 12 degree curve on the left. Chances are good that without the heel lifts we put in, their scoliosis would have gotten worse, especially T's. Consequently, with chiropractic care their necks healed better and their headaches went away. It is unfortunate they were never screened properly for scoliosis. If it had not been for the accident they never would have known they had a problem.

Remember, THERE WAS NO PAIN! It is important to implement regularly monitored scoliosis screenings throughout childhood and adolescence. Often pediatricians are too busy looking for serious diseases and monitoring internal health to be much help in examining children for back conditions. They usually see your children only when they are sick; however, this is not enough. The final responsibility belongs to the parents. You must watch your kids and be aware of the danger signs. After all, it is your child who suffers if a problem is not detected and corrected in time.

Although adults past their growing years are not primary candidates for scoliosis reduction, Dr. Charles Sallahian, D.C.[12] reports a case where a 45-year-old Caucasian male with a 22 degree curve right thoracic scoliosis came in for care. After three months of chiropractic management of his spine, new x-rays showed the lateral curves in his spine had been decreased to 16 degrees! The patient had a structural scoliosis and all thrusts into the spine were made against the convexities of the curves.

While there is no guarantee that all scoliosis patients will have as dramatic results as the above patients, it serves to remind us of the body's innate ability to heal itself given the proper environment. Further, not only did all of the above-mentioned patients have stronger, more flexible backs, but their symptoms decreased as well. Sometimes in the excitement of scientific improvement, we forget to acknowledge why the patient seeks care in the first place — relief of pain.

3

Back Pain—Why Does It Hurt and What Can Be Done About It?

The center of the universe is within us.

- David Amaral, D.C.

Now that you understand a little bit of the structure of the spine, we can talk about what goes wrong and causes it to hurt. First, we must explore the concept of pain and second, what exactly can chiropractic adjustment do for the subluxated spine. Spinal subluxation is when the vertebrae are out of their correct positions, creating a disturbance in the normal transmission of nerve energy.

Physiology of Pain

For the most part, pain is produced at the nerve endings by sensitive little structures known as nociceptors. When there is damage to tissue, for whatever reason, a substance is produced known as substance P. The nociceptors detect substance P and transmit the "pain" message to the brain. Ligaments, outer discs, facet joint capsules and other areas of the spine are loaded with these pain sensors. Nociceptors are in your back except in four areas: 1) the nucleus of the disc; 2) the inner annulus of the disc; 3) the articular cartilage of the facets and 4) ligamentum flauum. However, pain receptors may form in these structures if there is joint damage. Now you can appreciate the extreme sensitivity of the back to pain![13]

The Problem - Subluxation

Damage to the soft tissues surrounding a joint produces swelling. This in turn restricts the movement of the joint; nociceptors produce pain and may lead to muscle spasm. This is what a chiropractor calls a "subluxation." A "luxation" would be a total tearing of the joint; "sub" means "less than."

The Solution – The Adjustment

A controlled force introduced into the joint will increase the joint range of motion and break the spasm. This is a chiropractic adjustment (the medical term is manipulation of the spine). The adjustment acts as a counter-irritant by restoring motion, releasing endorphins, decreasing nociceptor stimulation and increasing mechanoreceptor (joint motion) firing. Adjusting the vertebrae also acts as a fluid pump which moves fresh synovial fluid through the joints of the spine. The adjustment usually produces a "pop" or audible sound which accompanies increased motion and reduced pain in the joint.

Malik Slosberg, M.S., D.C. of Life Chiropractic College West has his students try this simple test on themselves, which you may try if you wish. Select a finger and lightly pull on it to its normal end range. As you move the finger in and out, feel the end-play of the joint at the base of the finger. Now gently pull at the end range of motion until you "pop" the knuckle. This is known as cavitation.

The pop was the sound made as the gases in the joint expand out of solution causing a collapsing of the synovium. The synovium is the lining of the soft tissue between two structures which make a joint. Synovial fluid has gone into the joint. Like popping a champagne bottle cork, there has been an increase in amount and a decrease in pressure. Notice that you can now move your finger out further than before. There has been an expansion of the joint. This is what the chiropractor does to your spine. Just as the knuckle popping did not hurt, neither does this action hurt. Indeed, spinal adjustment will probably even feel good when done to the proper segments of the spine.

Reasons for Pain

Next, we'll look at ten reasons for pain in the back:

1. Trauma.

2. Poor posture.

3. Facet syndrome.

4. Disc problems.

5. Subluxated ribs.

6. Failed back surgery.

7. Common referred pain.

8. Scalenus Anticus syndrome.

9. Arthritis.

10. Direct trauma to the head.

1.   ***Trauma to the soft tissues/discs:*** What exactly is trauma? Trauma can essentially be broken down into two categories: macrotrauma and microtrauma. A good example of macrotrauma is a whiplash type of injury to your neck. This can result from a car accident, an impact to the head or face, falling backwards onto your head, bending over to lift something heavy without using good body mechanics, or falling from a ladder.

All these injuries could cause a serious disruption in the tissues. There could be a sudden tear or pull of the soft tissues away from the spine or other bones of the body. There may or may not be external bleeding. Almost surely there would be some bleeding on a microscopic level in the muscles, tendons, or ligaments. There would probably be swelling, redness, and heat over the area, as the body begins its normal healing response to this type of trauma.   This in turn would lead to fibrous adhesions, or scar tissue being formed. All of this causes PAIN!

The second type is called microtrauma. It is far more common and more easily overlooked. For example, microtrauma occurs when we hold our heads in a certain position for long periods of time, such as reading or watching television. By holding our heads forward, the muscles and ligaments in the back of the neck and the upper back must work harder and harder to keep the head in balance. This causes the same problems as macrotrauma. The tissue stretches and deforms (called plastic deformation) and will eventually scar as it tries to repair itself.

If you wish to experience what your upper back and neck muscles do all day long, try this experiment: take a 10-lb. weight and, while seated, hold the weight in your hand close to your shoulder with your elbow supported on the arm of a chair.   No problem, right? Now take your hand and hold the weight out away from your body. A little tougher, right? This is what happens when your head, which weighs about 15 lbs., moves out in front of your shoulders. You not only lose the natural neck curve, you build up tension in your neck and shoulders.

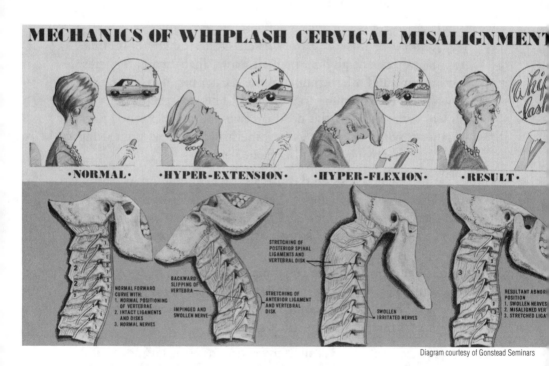

Diagram courtesy of Gonstead Seminars

This illustration shows how the neck goes from a normal position/curvature to an abnormal position/reverse curve during a whiplash injury. Often an x-ray is done to assess the damage.

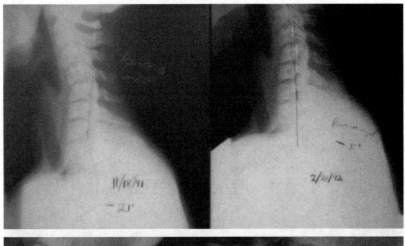

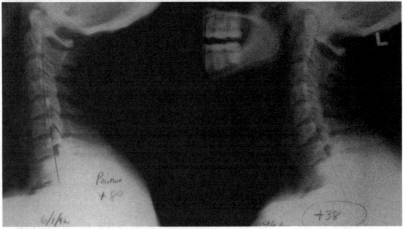

Correction of a whiplash with chiropractic care. Progressive correction for 11/18/91 (-21°) to 9/9/92 (+38°). Normal is 30°–60°.

The discs in your back are like little shock absorbers between the backbones, or vertebrae. They are extremely efficient and are made of fiber and cartilage.[14] The disc has two parts: the outside or fibrous rings, and the inside or nucleus pulposus. The outside is tough and hard, but the inside is soft and gelatinous, like toothpaste.

Everything goes fine until one day a too heavy load is suddenly transferred to the disc in a shearing motion (macrotrauma), or one side wears out by vertebrae pressing down on one side of

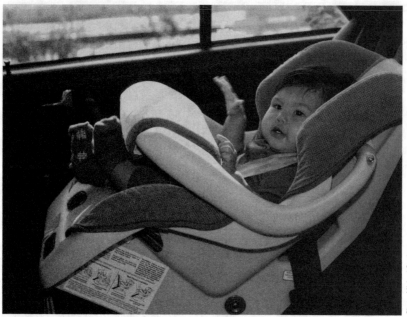

The best defense against whiplash and spinal trauma is to buckle-up at an early age. Here the child is belted to the car seat, which is belted to the back seat.

the disc more than the other for a long period of time (micro-trauma). A little of the "toothpaste" shoots out into the tough fibers of the disc rings, and the degeneration phase begins to accelerate. Patients often ask why I can't just put the disc back into the center where it belongs. Unfortunately, it is literally like trying to get toothpaste back into the tube!

One eventual result of trauma to the soft tissue is a process known as fibrosis of repair, commonly called scar tissue. This occurs as a result of the damaged tissue trying to repair itself as best it can.

Normal tissue is made up of a collagen matrix and is laid down in a crisscross pattern like a checkerboard. This tissue is soft, pliable and has a blood supply. After serious damage the tissue is torn on the microscopic level. Small "clean up" cells known as fibroclasts are sent by the body to eat away the destroyed collagen fibers.

Then the "builder" cells, known as fibroblasts, arrive and begin to rebuild with new collagen to replace what has been lost. The problem is that this new tissue is weaker, stiffer, less abundant, and less likely to lay down in the proper patterns as the old tissue. The new material is basically raw, weak tissue.

You might wonder how this new tissue can be made stronger? Tissue will lay itself down according to the stresses put on it. This is a concept known as "Wolfe's Law." The chiropractor's job is to help this process along by stressing the joint gently along the proper stress lines, so that the newly laid down tissue is close to the proper location and strength.

We do this by mobilizing and adjusting the joint in one direction, then doing deep transfrictional massage across the joint, ligament, tendon, or muscle in the other direction. This will stress the joint enough so that the new fibers are closer to their previous position. It will never be perfect, but it is much better than doing nothing.[15]

Another point about injured joints is that their own physiology begins to change. According to Malik Slosberg, M.S., D.C., injured joints begin to have a new sensory program that changes locally (peripheral nervous system), but also causes change at the spine (central nervous system). As a result of this occurring in the sensory area, the motor functions begin to change. An example of this is the antalgic, or sideways lean, of someone who is walking in pain. This can lead to a change in balance, coordination, and equilibrium. It may even cause nausea in someone who has had a severe injury to the neck.

This is why immobilization after an injury is often the worst thing which could be prescribed. Immobilization is good if there are broken bones or unstable ligaments around joints, but not good if there is simply stable soft tissue damage. When the joint is immobilized, messages from the joint to the spine and brain (proprioceptive input) are lost and the joint can be reinjured easily.

We know that immobilized joints, such as the facet joints of the spine, produce rapid degeneration of the articular facet cartilage. These joints do not have a blood supply. Rather, they receive their nutrition and release their waste by the flow of synovial fluid which is circulated by movement. Stasis of this fluid causes erosion and cracks in the membrane. When the chiropractor moves the vertebrae into their proper positions and restores proper movement, fresh synovial fluid is released into the joint. This is known as gapping the joint in a motion resembling a pump. The bottom line: motion is life!

2.   *Poor posture — muscular imbalance:*   One unique service your chiropractor can offer is a detailed analysis of your posture. As you learned in the last chapter, the spine when viewed from front to back is supposed to be straight. The pelvis should be level, based on two legs of even length; the spine should be straight, the shoulders level, and the head should sit on top of the neck with the eyes level to the horizon.

When viewed from the side, you should see normal kyphotic curves (located in the mid-back or thorax, and the tail bone-or-sacrum) and the normal lordotic curves (located in the neck or cervical region and the low back or lumbar region).

Most chiropractic techniques only look at the "Bone or Vertebrae-out-of-Place" theory. However, more and more chiropractors see posture as a direct indicator of a patient's health and internal condition. In all likelihood these doctors are working on the theories of Chiropractic Biophysics as developed by Dr. Don Harrison, who was mentioned in Chapter 2, along with his wife Dr. Sang Harrison, and his brother Dr. Glenn Harrison.

The Harrisons were not the first to look at postural faults, but they were the first to refine postural correction and elevate it to a science. Don systematically applied the principles of mathematics and physics to the spine and came up with equations and models which showed analysis and correction of the back could be more precise and more reproducible than ever thought before. In many cases if your chiropractor does not check your posture regularly, he or she may only be correcting part of your problem.

You can probably tell how it feels to walk around with bad posture and how much better it feels to have good posture. You stand straighter, are more relaxed, breathe deeper and easier, and generally move around more freely. The head is the end of a long lever—your spine. As your head moves either in front of or to the side of your body, you will feel the muscles and ligaments pull and stretch. You have created a lever which will get worse as your head moves further out of position. This will increase the amount of pain you feel as you walk or try to sit for long periods of time.

If the head is to one side of the body, you may experience pain over the hip area as more and more weight is forced onto the hips. This might make you think you have a hip problem when the real cause is your posture.

If you sit hunched over, your mid-back may cause you pain and you might feel the need to stretch upright. Your breathing may also diminish as the internal organs of the chest are crushed forward by the weight put on them. Even the heart may be adversely affected.

The spinal cord is of finite length. As the head moves forward or to the side, stress is added to the nerves as they move down the sides and out the spine. Postural adjusting restores the natural structure and decreases the length of the spinal cord. As the cervical curve comes back, according to the work made famous by Alf Breig, M.D., there will be less stress on the cervical spinal cord and less pressure on the nerves as they exit the spine on the sides.[16]

If poor posture is not corrected, the nerves which are under stress as they exit the spine will eventually scar over and begin to lose their function. Each nerve has its own tiny blood supply system. The health of the nerve is dependent on the circulation of blood to keep it oxygenated and fed with nutrients and free of waste products. One result of stretching due to bad posture is that blood vessels become damaged and cannot deliver the proper amount of blood. Eventually the nerve cells die or become dysfunctional.

Very few health disciplines look at the broad spectrum of your body, integrating ideas and problems which cause dis–ease. Those that don't, have philosophies based on a reductionist model which reduces the painful area down to its respective molecular structures. This is fine when a chemical problem exists, or a biochemical disorder is suspected; however, it may be way off base when the problem is structural or mechanical.

If you had been poisoned, clearly a chemical problem, you would not go to a chiropractor. Rather you would go to an M.D. who would give you a chemical solution, i.e., a drug or antidote, which would neutralize the poison. A chiropractor would address your back problem, which to you is most commonly pain, and determine if a biomechanical fault, such as posture or misaligned vertebrae, exists and adjust it back into its proper position. A chemical problem requires a chemical solution, and a mechanical problem requires a mechanical solution.

B.J. Palmer, the prominent son of the founder of chiropractic, said that a specialist is someone who knows more and more about less and less. Chiropractors, for the most part, try to integrate other areas of the patient's life into the health care plan. In reality, chiropractors have been criticized for trying to advise patients on the importance of diet, positive mental outlook, proper exercise, and a good night's sleep. All of these factors contribute to

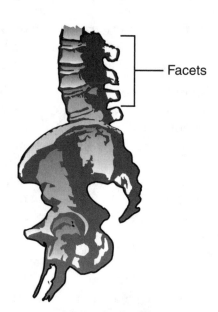

— Facets

Facets in the low back may compress causing low back pain. In the latter stages of pregnancy or in the case of a large tummy, the stress on the facets is greater. This is known as facet syndrome.

chiropractic management by helping adjustments hold better and last longer.

We are trying to incorporate a whole life approach to your health. Imagine a new model of health, specifically one in which the main focus is health, not disease or sickness. We call this the "wellness model" and encourage our patients to focus on and move toward this goal. There will be more on this later.

3.   *Facet syndrome:*   The vertebral facets are four small joints (two each in two sets) located in the back of each vertebra. They interlock with the vertebrae directly above and below to form a joint complex and allow for mobility. They are located throughout the entire spine but are angled differently in different parts of the spine. The facets are what make the "popping" sound when the chiropractor adjusts your back as they stretch back into their proper position.

Facets also perform one other major function: along with the discs, they form the opening of the hole through which the nerve exits in the side of the spine. This hole is called the intervertebral foramina (IVF). Unlike the discs, there is no fiber between the facets, only a soft substance known as synovial membrane.[17] Facets are directly connected to the nervous system, and when compressed they feel PAIN!

The back has many curves and angles to it. Some are there by design, others are not. The facets may jam against each other causing pain. Thus, they need to be stretched and loosened. Certain types of traction are helpful, but the best way to unlock the joint effectively is to manipulate or adjust it.

Only a chiropractor is fully trained to do this correctly. In some states only chiropractors may legally adjust the spine. The reasons are simple: many health professionals such as M.D.s, physical therapists, and others can get the joint to go "pop," but only a chiropractor has spent four years in school and many years in practice perfecting the art of adjusting. Adjusting is not just shoving on the spine to hear a click, but rather moving one or more vertebrae in a specific direction with a specific force to a specific depth. It takes years to learn this.

It is most important to know which joint or series of joints to adjust and which ones to leave alone. Osteopaths formerly were trained extensively in manipulation techniques, medicine, and surgery, but now usually only work with medications and surgery, having given up spinal manipulation in favor of more invasive procedures. Chiropractors are the best in the world at manipulating or adjusting the joints of the spine.

Chiropractors make a point of differentiating a manipulation which someone (other than a chiropractor) may perform to mobilize a stuck joint, such as a vertebra, from a chiropractic "adjustment." A chiropractic adjustment has subtle differences and is often distinguished by whatever technique the chiropractor uses. In all cases, there is a reduction of tension in the nervous system, more mobility in the joints, and a return of the body to a more normal physiologic state.

For example, if the practitioner does motion palpation adjusting (adjusting the spine precisely where there is a loss of spinal mobility) there will be less resistance in the joint to fixation and better mobility once the adjustment has been made.

If the practitioner utilizes upper cervical adjusting (C1, C2), such as Biophysics, Toggle, NUCCA, Grostic or Sweat Techniques, there will be a reduction of tension in the brain stem as it exits the skull. This will cause the entire body to work in a more efficient state. The immune system will be directly improved, as will the amount of blood delivered to the organs of the body.[18]

This is because the sympathetic nervous system controls the amount of blood which reaches the organs of our bodies. The more blood that reaches our organs, the more oxygen those organs receive. More oxygen produces better tissue health. This means your internal organs will function better and last longer.

Once the facets have been opened up or adjusted, the pain begins to subside almost immediately. If there has been any direct pressure on the nerve either by the bone or the soft tissue surrounding the facets, there should be an immediate reduction of this pressure. Consequently, any malfunction of that nerve arising from pressure would also be relieved and the organ, gland, or muscle at the end of the nerve would begin to function as its original intention. You are interested in the pain going away quickly. Your chiropractor wants that as well, but more importantly, he or she wants your general health to get better, not just stopping your back pain.

If the facets begin to grow larger due to stress, bone pathology or trauma, (hypertrophy) then the hole the nerve passes through will become smaller. This is known as foraminal stenosis. It may also be caused by misaligned vertebrae, which cause swelling and put pressure on the nerve.

"Pinching" on the nerve may result in localized pain and possibly radiating pain down into the arms or hands (if the problem exists in the neck) or into the legs or feet (if the problem exists in the low back). An adjustment should relieve this last condition; however, if there is permanent bone growth and the canal has become smaller, it may be necessary to have surgery known as a foraminotomy. Such surgery should be your last alternative.

Chiropractic adjustments, traction, physical therapy, and even acupuncture are the least invasive measures and entail the least amount of risk. If these fail, your chiropractor may consult with a medical specialist for possible drug therapy, such as anti-inflammatory medications and painkillers in conjunction with the adjustments, depending on your case and his or her philosophy. If all else fails, an operation may be the only answer.

4.   *Disc problems:*   I have referred to the discs previously as small shock absorber pads which live between the vertebrae. They act as a cushion for the vertebrae to rest on, absorbing compressive blows to the spine and allowing a pivot point for bending, flexing and rotating the body. Unfortunately, there are many things which can go wrong with the discs. They may be damaged by trauma or become worn out by time and overuse. It is the most common cause of back pain, and the one condition feared by most people. The disc looks like a ball bearing in the center of a very thick phonographic record and consists of two parts.

Annular Rings: The annular rings are the outside of the disc. They are tough, fibrous and have much resiliency to resist the torquing motion of the spine as we bend and twist. The fibers of the annulus are arranged in three different configurations. One layer is oriented so that the fibers run straight up and down. The next layer angles to the right; the final layer angles to the left. This pattern promotes and provides strength in all directions for bending. It also allows maximum strength and flexibility.

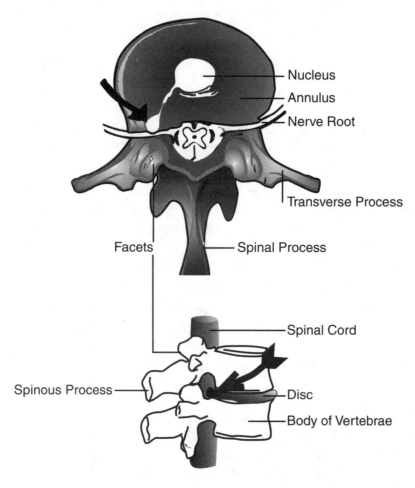

Disc in both top view (top picture) and side view (bottom picture). In both cases the arrow points to a nucleus protrusion.

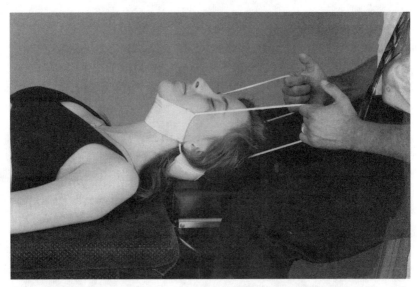

Super Traction. Here, a doctor gently pulls and holds constant tension on the neck for 30 seconds to two minutes. This technique is used for herniated cervical discs.

Nucleus Pulposus: The nucleus is the inside of the disc and resists compression, that is the force of gravity straight down on the spine. The nucleus resembles a ball bearing or ball of toothpaste. As long as the compressive forces do not exceed the load capability of the nucleus, you are in fine shape. Yet the nucleus is only as strong as the annular rings. If one or more begins to rupture, the nuclear contents will start to leak out, usually towards the spinal cord.

Let's look at some regions of the spine and how damaged discs affect each area. Many things cause discs to deteriorate, including trauma, bad posture, scoliosis, subluxations and work hazards such as improper sitting or lifting.

Cervical Disc: Bad cervical discs are very rare when compared to lumbar discs. In my office I see approximately 100 lumbar discs to one cervical disc. First, a quick anatomy lesson (groan!). In the back of the vertebral bodies from your head to your tail bone is a very strong ligament called the posterior longitudinal ligament (PLL). This ligament is stronger and wider at the top by the neck than at the bottom by the lumbars. Consequently, discs are being held in place better at the top.

In addition, there is only the head's weight on the discs of the neck, while there is the weight of the entire upper body on the discs of the lumbars. Finally, in the neck, the discs are held tightly in place by little "lips" called uncinate processes, which are absent in the low back. For all these reasons, there is less likelihood of a disc problem in the cervicals than in the lower back.

When a patient has the symptoms of a problem with a cervical disc, it can be the result of a sudden trauma, years of minor abuse (such as having the head forward of the shoulders all the time) or the result of a congenital malformation or birth defect. It is also likely to be a fairly serious case, since the spinal cord at the cervical level is very close to the brain stem.

Some signs and symptoms of a cervical disc problem are pain, numbness, tingling radiating from the neck down the arms and into the hands, pain radiating down from the neck into the middle of the shoulder blade, or pain in the neck which increases as the patient coughs, sneezes, or strains at the stool. Depending on which level of the spinal cord is involved, there are varying symptoms which the doctor looks for. Stanley Hoppenfield, M.D.'s excellent book, *Orthopaedic Neurology—A Diagnostic Guide to Neurologic Levels* is one of the best texts in the field today that explains cervical disc problems.[19]

Care of a cervical disc lesion is rather varied in its approach. The chiropractor may elect to do more traction and only minimal adjusting. According to Daniel Murphy, D.A.B.C.O., who lectures extensively on whiplash trauma, adjusting the cervical disc may sometimes make it worse. Depending on the severity of the disc bulge, adjusting the site of the lesion may cause the disc to be "squished around" by the uncinate processes (the aforementioned "lips").

Traction, especially what Dr. Murphy calls "super traction," will have the most benefit. Super traction is manual traction by the chiropractor where the head is slowly tractioned to its greatest elongation by means of a special harness, then held in place for a few seconds. The idea is to create a pseudo vacuum in which the herniated disc material (the nucleus) is slightly suctioned back into place. Next, interferential current using microamperage is used on the neck across the damaged area in order to create a healing effect on the outside of the disc or the annular rings. This method seems to work well if there has not been too much damage to the disc.

A medical doctor will probably recommend corticosteroids, and a surgeon will probably want to do surgery. Steroids may cause death of the tissue in the neck by disrupting the blood supply. The proteoglycans (a type of protein which acts as cement in the disc) become dried out and water is driven out of the joint. This condition is not reversible. Remember, once you have surgery, you can never replace what has been cut out, so consider it only as a last resort.

A damaged cervical disc may be a dismal prognosis. The best approach is to get more than one opinion and as many good diagnostic tests as possible. Always start with the most conservative therapy offered — usually chiropractic. If that isn't working, ask the chiropractor to help you find a good medical doctor. If medicine doesn't work, surgery may be the only alternative. Throughout it all, even post-surgically, you may still be adjusted in the other levels of your spine, especially non-force specific adjusting to the C1 atlas. In this way, your healing time will be lessened because your nervous system will work better overall.

Thoracic Disc: Thoracic disc problems are fairly rare. When they do occur, they are often the result of severe trauma to the spine, such as a fall in which you land on your feet and compress the spine. The vertebrae may burst or the discs may break themselves apart. If the patient has a severe kyphosis, a hunching forward of the shoulders and back, there may be compression in the front of the vertebral bodies and discs. The discs may degenerate early in the front at an accelerated rate. This might cause a thoracic disc problem.

Lumbar Disc: According to the *Merck Manual*,[20] 80% of degenerated lumbar disc problems are in the L5-S1 area and affect the L5 or S1 nerve roots. Lumbar disc pain is the foremost cause of low back pain today and keeps millions of people from living a normal, pain-free life.

As the disc degenerates, the nucleus of the disc usually moves backwards through the normally tough fibers of the outer rings. With each new trauma, the rings tear either all at once or a little at a time. The push towards the spinal cord is known as posterior (towards the back of the body) protrusion. The disc may push straight back into the spinal cord or may push posterolaterally (backwards and to the sides) and compress the nerve roots as they exit the spinal cord. This produces major PAIN and may cause the classic sciatica, or pain down the leg. *(see diagram pg. 58)*

The disc may deteriorate so badly that it squishes and flows (like toothpaste) around the posterior longitudinal ligament (PLL). This ligament stretches from the top of the spine down to the tip of the tailbone at the coccyx and is designed to keep the discs in their place. If the disc material moves around this ligament and presses against a nerve or the spinal cord, it is known as a prolapsed disc. These are very difficult to treat.

In fact, if part of the disc moves around the PLL, and then is pinched off by the outside of the disc trying to heal and protect itself, it may leave that part of the nucleus "floating" around the spinal cord. Thus, there may be a multitude of symptoms as the fragment moves around, or it may lodge somewhere and cause no symptoms at all.

If a disc is simply bulging into the spinal cord, the chiropractor or medical doctor will observe how you walk into the clinic. If you are leaning away from the painful side, then you have what is known as a lateral disc bulge. That is, the disc is bulging such that the nerves which lead to the sciatic nerve are towards the inside or medial aspect of the disc. This is called an antalgic lean away from the disc. When you lean your body this way, you are pulling the nerves away from the discs. When this pressure is relieved the pain is reduced or eliminated. If the disc problem is bad enough, there may be protrusion into the hole known as the intervertebral foramina from which the nerve exits.

If you are leaning toward the painful side of your back or leg, then you probably have a medial disc protrusion. Here the disc is bulging such that the nerves which lead to the sciatic nerve are towards the outside or lateral of the spinal cord. As you lean toward the painful side, you are again pulling the nerves away from the discs. This will reduce the pain.

Occasionally, a disc may protrude to the center of the spinal cord. When this happens, the patient will probably lean forward in a flexed position in order to relieve the pressure of the nerves on the disc. If the disc damage is severe enough, it may not only affect the nerves leading to the sciatic nerve but also compress the sacral nerve roots.

This is a serious situation. There may be a condition known as foot drop, where the foot actually falls when trying to take a step, or there may be paralysis of the bladder or bowel. If you are totally incontinent—either cannot go to the bathroom or cannot make it to the bathroom, you may have a condition known as cauda equina syndrome. The cauda equina is the end of the spinal cord and is an important area if there is nerve pressure. This is usually a medical emergency and may require immediate surgery to relieve the pressure before permanent damage results.

Definitive diagnosis can sometimes be made with plain film x-rays, although in many cases the chiropractor or medical doctor may order a CAT scan (Computerized Axial Tomography) or an MRI (Magnetic Resonance Imaging) or even a myelogram, where a dye is injected into the disc and then x-rayed.

The myelogram is more invasive and dangerous than the other tests and may not be diagnostically superior. The difference between the CAT scan and the MRI is that the CAT scan uses a lot of radiation but is the best for seeing bony problems. The MRI uses powerful magnets and no radiation to make an image. The MRI is superior for showing soft tissue lesions such as disc protrusion and nerve impingement (compression).

Chiropractic adjusting is always very specific, but especially so when is a disc involved. As with the cervical disc, the chiropractor may not do a typical low back adjustment. Often he or she will use lumbar flexion and distraction adjustments. This means the patient is lying on the stomach in a flexed position. The doctor will then stretch the low back in order to pump the disc with fluid. This would be contraindicated if the disc is "hot", that is, already very swollen and painful.

The chiropractor may also use "Cox Technique," where a combination of the patient's breathing, spinal flexion, traction and lifting on the spinous process of the vertebrae involved will help to relieve the pressure on the disc. This method is extremely effective and has kept many patients out of surgery. The chiropractor may use flexion; side posture adjusting known as Diversified Techniques. Usually any type of flexing or flexion adjusting will relieve low back pain. When there is a disc involved, it must be done GENTLY!

5.   *Subluxated Ribs:* R was lifting a heavy computer monitor when he felt something "pop" in his midback. He was lifting correctly from the floor to his waist by using his legs and not straining his back. Unfortunately, he forgot to exhale as he lifted, and the force of his full lungs and the increased pressure as he lifted caused one of his ribs to displace slightly. The pain was sharp, immediate, slightly to the side of the spine, and radiated around to the front of his chest.

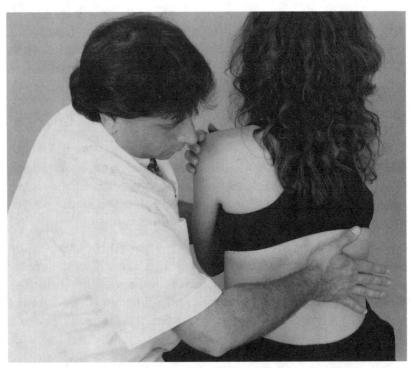

Here the chiropractor sets a lower rib with the patient in a seated position.

It took two adjustments to fix this problem. It probably would have been worse had he not come in right away because scar tissue would have formed around the joint and caused many painful adhesions. Usually the longer the rib is out of its natural alignment, the longer it takes to stabilize.

In the back, the rib heads connect to the body of the vertebrae as they cross the transverse process. They connect with the vertebra above, the vertebra below, and the disc between them. However, the first and the last three ribs only connect with their own vertebral body. Subluxations of the first rib by the base of the neck can cause many problems including pain and numbness down an arm, as these compress the nerves.

Breathing too deeply and holding the breath too long or any extreme motion which pulls the arm back behind the body in a sudden jerking motion can also cause ribs to subluxate. Dr. Darrell Lavin of Castro Valley, California takes care of many baseball players (he himself was a pitcher for the University of California at Santa Barbara) and says he treats many outfielders who catch balls just out of their reach or behind them.

Weight lifting can cause the ribs to subluxate if the weight is too great or the breathing is improper. Wrestling and tackle football are more direct causes of knocking ribs out of place, and rib fractures are often caused as well.

The adjustment is fairly simple. The chiropractor will use either a drop table, activator (a hand-held instrument), or some efficient lever to quickly "pop" the rib back into its proper position. Usually there is very little force, but the adjustment must be made precisely and quickly or it may hurt a little. Total relaxation on the part of the patient is absolutely essential.

6.   *Failed back surgery:* It is truly unfortunate that more people do not seek chiropractic care before they allow themselves to be put under the knife. I would go one step further and say their medical doctor should automatically recommend a consultation with a chiropractor before surgery, unless it is a medical emergency. I might even make the suggestion that it is medical

malpractice not to recommend a consultation with a good chiropractor before proceeding with surgery.

The basis for my statements is recent research that indicates chiropractic patients do exceptionally well when compared to medical patients with the same type of back problem, in all but the most serious cases. This is demonstrated by fewer lost days of work, less chronic pain, less costly treatment, and greater patient satisfaction.[21]

A State of Washington Workers' Compensation study reported that two years after fusion back surgery, 68% of the patients were still work disabled and 23% required further lumbar surgery.[22] If 91 out of 100 cases are not helped, what are your chances for success with back surgery?

Then why aren't more M.D.s prescribing or recommending chiropractic care for their patients? What matters is that the patient gets well. If it is malpractice for the chiropractor to fail to send the patient to an M.D. if the patient needs medical attention, then doesn't the same standard apply if the patient might benefit from chiropractic care? Medical doctors may argue that physical therapists are doing what chiropractors do, but it is chiropractic care which is getting the positive results in the studies done today.

The truth is that no one can do what a chiropractor does except a chiropractor. Truly bright medical people do not see chiropractic as a threat or a danger. Rather, they are intensely curious about what the chiropractor knows and what different perspectives the D.C. can offer. These medical doctors only want the best for their patients and seem to have few economic concerns or personal egos to maintain.

Most people will tell you that you should usually try the more conservative therapies first. This is especially true in the care of the back. According to Stanley Bigos, M.D., only 7% of patients with a bad back have true radiculopathy (irritation of nerve roots that cause pain, numbness or tingling down the legs or arms), and a diskectomy (removal of the disc) is only good for 2% of patients. This means that 98% of current patients undergoing disc removal surgery may be receiving ineffective treatment![23]

Chiropractic care is the most conservative, safe and natural therapy available and should be tried first. If this doesn't work, an M.D. should try mild drugs in combination with chiropractic and physical therapy. If that still doesn't work, then a battery of diagnostic tests are performed such as MRI's, CAT scans, and nerve conduction studies. They may even try steroid injections, although this may not have any benefit, and may lead to permanent damage to the joint.

Finally, medical doctors may say that surgery is the only answer. What you must understand is that after bone is removed to relieve the pressure and pain on the nerves, there may eventually be a regrowth of scar tissue on the surgery site that will replace the removed bone. Bear in mind that only 2%–9% are successful.

It is important to realize that the body is a lot smarter than we give it credit. When bone is removed from the back, the body will try to replace it with something else. The only thing the body has to work with is fibrous scar tissue produced by cells called fibroblasts. This scar tissue is tough and hard. It may start to compress again on the nerves where the bone was removed earlier.

The surgery may also change the configuration of the back, making it curve where it didn't curve before, or taking out a curve that was there previously. When this occurs the tiny electric charges in the back will change.[24] Just as with scoliosis curves, the areas in the back that are now under more stress will have a slightly negative charge. This will attract calcium which is positively charged. Opposites attract and the calcium will be laid down in this area as new bone. This will further increase the pressure on the nerves.

It should be obvious that as bone is removed from the back, it changes the way the back works. Increased pressure is added to areas where there was little or no pressure before, and pressure is decreased on structures which are specifically designed to support the back. According to Malik Slosberg, M.S., D.C. of Life Chiropractic College West, the problem with fusing L5-S1 is that within three to four years a high percentage of L4-L5 discs herniate. This is due to the increased amount of stress placed on that disc.

According to one study,[25] discs without pumping action due to increased loads showed marked degenerative joint disease. Under high forces, the disc can become very acidic and increase its metabolic enzymes. These waste products are not driven out when the pumping action is ceased. Essentially, the intervertebral disc lives because of changing pressures and movement. Absent these forces, it degenerates.

Thus, with surgery the back will move and work differently—often less efficiently. A simple analogy is to take a skyscraper in any major city, or a bridge such as the Golden Gate, and knock out a few of the major walls and structures that support it. Then as it starts to lean, shake, or bend, send in a crew of construction people. They can do anything they want except one thing: replace the walls that were taken out as they were originally constructed. The structure will never be the same, will it? It may continue to stand, but if an earthquake or a strong wind comes up, watch out! Similarly, if the post-surgical patient puts his or her back under an abnormal load, as occurs in sports, lifting, sitting or good old-fashioned stress, it is likely to fail.

Other reasons for failed back surgery may simply be that doctors are only human. There have been decompression cases (removal of bone from compressed nerves) where the wrong level of the spine has been operated on. Too much bone may have been removed or not enough. The scalpel or other sharp instrument may nick or sever the spinal nerves. The anesthetic may cause damage to the nerves or even kill the patient. Chymopapain, an enzyme derived from papaya that is sometimes injected into the spine to shrink a bulging disc, may eat away at the healthy part of the disc and cause early degeneration. The patient may even be allergic to the enzyme, or it might have been injected at the wrong level. The point is that anything can go wrong in surgery and often does.

Donald R. Murphy, D.C. cites several factors to explain why back surgeries fail in the first place.[26] First, the patient may have been misdiagnosed and may not need surgery at all. He cites Kirkaldy-Willis and Tilscher by saying that 90-97% of all back pain is due to dysfunction of either the spinal joints or the muscles or both.[27]

A second problem with low back surgeries, according to Dr. Murphy, is that many muscles of the back can cause pain and spasticity when they develop trigger points as described in other parts of this text. Third, there is the problem of the subluxation-complex as described by chiropractors.

One issue which has been discussed recently in back surgery circles is the concept of pain derived from the chiropractic subluxation. Many surgeons agree that pain is caused from the back being subluxated or misaligned. They also agree that the spine may become subluxated during surgery, and they have no way of identifying this while the patient is on the table. This has caused some surgeons and patients to request that a chiropractor be in the operating room during the procedure to adjust and align the spine while the patient's back is still open, or direct the surgeon to do it.

The next step may be to fuse that part of the back together to give it stability so the back will not be locked into subluxation. This treatment is by no means widespread at this point, but as more and more chiropractors are gaining hospital privileges, it is becoming increasingly popular. It is also nice to see the two professions working together for the benefit of everyone.

Another procedure which is gaining some acceptance is known as manipulation under anesthesia (also known as "Manipulation Under Seation Treatment"–"MUST"). This is when chiropractic manipulation ("adjustment") is done on an anesthetized patient who cannot be adjusted when awake. The reasons may be extensive scar tissue in post-surgical sites, areas of extensive trauma, osteoarthritis, or some chronically inflamed areas. An anesthesiologist puts the patient under light anesthesia which relaxes skeletal muscle and blocks pain. Once the patient is asleep, two chiropractors move the patient into position and manipulate the problem area. The patient is then taken into the recovery room for approximately one hour. This procedure is generally done on an outpatient basis and may need to be repeated

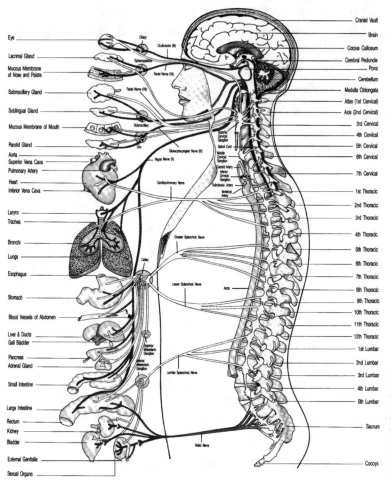

Diagram courtesy of The Parker Foundation

Autonomic Nervous System. The part of the nervous system which affects the viscera (organs) of the body.

two or three times.   Sometimes the chiropractic manipulations are also combined with physical therapy sessions. These new procedures provide renewed hope for many chronic pain patients, while forging new alliances between the professions.

If you have already had back surgery, a chiropractor will do a detailed examination of your present condition. Your surgery record will be looked at carefully in order to determine exactly what the surgeon performed. Changes in the anatomy can be dealt with, but we have to know just what we are dealing with. Once we have determined what the problem is and how it may be resolved, a course of care can be developed for you.

7.   ***Common Referred Pain:*** Many times you will tell your doctor of chiropractic that you hurt in a certain spot and he or she will adjust you somewhere else. You may wonder why they would do that. If you say there is pain over your shoulder blade, the doctor of chiropractic may check your gallbladder or your neck.   Pain running down the left arm could indicate neck problems, shoulder problems, or even the classic pain syndrome of a myocardial infarction or heart attack. These are all examples of what is known as referred pain—that is, pain whose origin is at one place in the body but is felt at another part of the body.

This is one of the main reasons you should see a chiropractor. You never know what may be causing these aches and pains you are feeling. It may be something as small as a strained muscle or some other minor symptom. However, it could be something crucial and should be explored.

The body is put together in an extremely complex way. Many sciences and therapies are emerging based on this concept; one example is reflexology and another is acupressure. Both work on the principle that positive therapies can be accomplished by working on other sites in the body. Concerning the back, there are many problems with the body which refer pain to the back. They fall into two categories:

Visceral: The word "viscera" means that organs are involved—the heart, lungs, stomach, kidneys, or other organs. These organs do not have the classic pain fibers that the back possesses. They transmit a pain-like sensation (such as an upset stomach), but very often it goes unnoticed. However, what they may do is transmit the pain to the spine via a group of nerves known as the sympathetic ganglion fibers, which are a part of the autonomic nervous system.

An example of this is the gallbladder. When the gallbladder is full of calcium deposits, known as stones, it may send pain signals

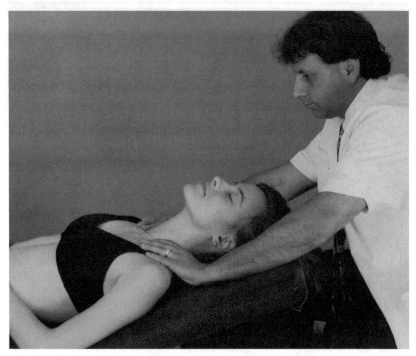

Muscle work on the scalene muscles at the side and base of the neck. These muscles become extremely tight, especially if your occupation involves sitting and leaning the head forward. Secretaries, nurses, computer workers, etc. are susceptible to this.

to the lower part of the shoulder blade, usually on the right side. Another example of a more immediate nature is that of a heart attack. A patient may complain of upper back and shoulder pain long before the crushing sensation in the chest indicates that they are having an attack.

Again, this is why it is so important to be examined by your chiropractor. As I tell my patients, you may be out playing golf or swinging a tennis racket and feel that sudden pain between your shoulder blades. It could be your heart or it could be your back. Plus, if it is your back, those nerves which are compressed and are causing the pain do go to your heart and lungs. Yes, you can live with a sore back but can you afford to overlook the organs which keep you alive?

Somatic: The word "soma" means body, and in this case refers to the musculoskeletal system, that is the muscles, tendons, ligaments, and bones. Many times it may hurt at one level of the spine, but in reality the problem is elsewhere. Classically, there may be pain in one of the extremities such as your wrist, and the problem is really in your neck. The reason I say classic is because of the significance the wrist has for people, especially those who enjoy using their hands. Problems of the wrist are often lumped under the heading of "carpal tunnel syndrome." However, the pressure on the nerve may not be in the wrist at all, but rather where the nerve leaves the neck. There will be more on this in the chapter pertaining to the extremities.

8.   *Scalenus Anticus Syndrome* — What??: Scalenus Anticus muscle syndrome is one of the most overlooked and easily treatable dysfunctions that can occur in the neck. The scalene muscles are on the side of the neck. They are used and overused daily during many movements. For example, any pulling that is done by the arm from front to back, such as a supermarket checker might do, could cause the muscles to overwork, get larger (hypertrophy) and cause some compression on the nerves going into the hand.

The nerves which go into the hands (the brachial plexus), pass under the scalenes and go into the arm. As the muscle gets bigger, it may shut off the flow of nerve impulses into the hand and cause numbness, tingling, pain and coldness (if the artery is involved), probably in that order.

Donald Murphy, D.C. says that when the scalene muscles develop trigger points they can refer pain not only into the thumb and the index finger, but also into the chest, shoulder, the back and sides of the arms, and even to the medial or inside edge of the shoulder blade.[28] It may even imitate the symptoms of carpal tunnel syndrome. Therefore, it is important for your doctor to examine this thoroughly, prior to any therapy on the wrist itself.

Adjusting the neck may help if there is a problem with the vertebrae and nerve roots, but one of the most effective therapies for this disorder is something called "spray and stretch." Spray and stretch uses a very cold volatile substance which freezes the muscles and allows the doctor to actually stretch the tissues beyond their normal pain tolerance. This causes a "slackening" of the normally tight fibers which are constricting the nerve sheath. This loosening of the tissue will cause a decrease in the pressure on the nerves.

In addition, your doctor of chiropractic may also perform or prescribe deep friction tissue massage and trigger point therapy to try and loosen the tissue.[29] This should help your symptoms improve, but if the pressure has been there a long time, do not expect an overnight miracle; it may take some time.

9.   *Arthritis:*   Often patients tell me they feel their pain is a result of "old age." I ask them what they mean by old age and they say the things that happen to everyone such as arthritis, as if it's a birthright. I tell them that old age does not necessarily mean guaranteed pain, and I mean this. Usually it takes only a few adjustments before they believe me, but chiropractors can almost always get people out of pain.

Arthritis simply means inflammation in the joints. Since inflammation is usually painful, arthritis is usually painful. Inflammation occurs when the joint is overused or abnormal pressure or stress is put upon it. Arthritis can occur wherever there is a joint in the body. Different types of arthritis will affect different regions of the body. I will limit our discussion to two major types of arthritis.

Degenerative: Degenerative arthritis is also known as osteoarthritis ("osteo" means bone). Due to a loss of the shock absorbing pad (a synovial membrane made of hyaline cartilage) between the two bones that form the joint, the bones are closer to each other than they should be. This causes them to grind bone on bone and wear out faster as they are used. This causes inflammation and lots of pain.

According to the *Merck Manual*,[30] osteoarthritis (OA) is seen universally in all vertebrates, primarily in weight-bearing joints. This suggests it is really more the body's repair process in response to adverse pressure than a disease. It is even seen in animals that have their weight supported by water, such as dolphins and whales, but not in animals which hang upside down, such as bats and sloths.

There are many causes of this process, most of which are unknown, yet we do see a genetic disposition towards degeneration. Other factors such as infection and neurological or vascular problems may be causes. Trauma to a joint, such as when vertebrae are knocked out of their normal position by some force and have restricted motion, is a likely cause.

What happens to the joint is that the hyaline cartilage becomes damaged, and the tissue that replaces the healthy synovial membrane is scar tissue inside and around the joint. It is weaker, more brittle and more sensitive. This may eventually take the form of little bone spurs which look like spikes around the joint. The fluid which is normally inside the joint begins to leak out and does not return without proper rest, specific mobility and exercise to the area.

Many times OA will go unnoticed because it does not hurt until the problem has advanced. Early signs are stiffness in the morning or following inactivity which gets better with motion and pain which gets worse with vigorous exercise. As time goes on without proper care, you can expect things to get worse. The joint wears out and gets stiffer and more painful. The ligaments surrounding the joint become lax and cause more instability and increased pain. Injuries are more likely with daily activities. In the neck and the low back, there is a chance the pain will radiate into the arms or down the legs as the nerve roots are affected by the degeneration.

The chiropractor will try to keep the joints mobile with adjustments but may also give exercises to enhance mobility and develop stress-absorbing tendons and muscles, along with stretches to do on your own. You will be encouraged to rest at appropriate times to allow the cartilage to rehydrate as much as possible. You will be instructed to avoid soft chairs and beds and perform postural exercises to minimize abnormal wear on the joints. As long as the vertebrae are in proper alignment, the wear on the discs will be reduced and distributed more evenly.

Rheumatoid: Rheumatoid arthritis (RA) is in the classification of diseases known as "autoimmune disorders." This means that the body is attacking itself in some way. This disorder is usually chronic and is characterized by symmetric inflammation of the peripheral joints. This disorder is different from OA mentioned above. Whereas OA is characterized by a loss of synovial membrane between the joints, RA is characterized by an increase in this tissue. The membrane folds and thickens, causing an increase in joint size and a change in the articulation or movement of the joint. Other responses of the body include a combination of fibrosis, necrosis (death), and erosion of tissue in the joint.

Patients feel pain in the inflamed joints and often see the swelling in the same joint on each side of the body (as seen in the small joints of the hand, wrists, elbows and ankles). Stiffness in the morning or after inactivity may last 30 minutes or more. Unlike OA, rheumatoid arthritis is usually diagnosed easily with laboratory and x-ray findings.

Conservative management such as chiropractic adjustments to help the neurology and passive motion to help the symptoms is usually recommended. In a study done by Toshima Yamauchi, M.D., et al., rheumatism occurs at night when there is little or no movement in the joints.[31] This leads to a decrease in the circulation of synovial fluid and a decrease in the pH (increase of acidity) in the joint. The authors found passive slow motion to the affected joint at night was better than no motion.

Although the Merck Manual makes an issue out of being careful about diet therapy and "quackery," John A. McDougall, M.D. draws some important conclusions in the relationship between diet and arthritis.[32] He cites people in Africa, Japan and China, with lifestyles and dietary customs different from Americans, who have very few instances of RA. Unlike the United States, where animal fat is a major part of our diet and we have an incidence of 1% to 4% of Americans suffering from RA, these people consume very few animal products; the diet is basically starch-centered (complex carbohydrate). However, when these people are moved to the United States and/or adopt a rich

Western diet, rheumatoid arthritis becomes as common with them as it does with Americans.

Dr. McDougall cites several studies which show how diet plays an important role in the cause and care of RA patients. He tells of a study done at Wayne State University Medical School where six RA patients were fed a fat-free diet. Within seven weeks all six were in complete remission from RA. The symptoms recurred within seventy-two hours when animal fats or vegetable oil were consumed by the patients.

Dr. McDougall adds to the conclusions of the investigators by noting that the elimination of cheese and meat from their diet probably made a major contribution to the remission. His reasoning is that dairy products and meats are common sources of the antibodies which enter the bloodstream and joints, form an irritant, and then are attacked by the antibodies of the immune system.

If you have known food allergies and suffer from RA, stay away from these foods. Also, if you have RA, you would probably benefit from a diet low in fats and proteins and high in complex carbohydrates. For further information, pick up a copy of *McDougall's Medicine* at your local bookstore.

10. *Direct Trauma to the Head:* When a person has sustained direct trauma to the head, there are many things to consider. One obvious threat is bleeding under the skull next to the brain. This is known as a subdural hematoma and is a medical emergency in most cases. The surgeon will open the skull and relieve the pressure. Then the site of the bleeding will be cauterized or closed to prevent future problems. In my pre-chiropractic years working as an anesthesia tech in surgery, I observed and participated in many of these operations. This type of care is obviously beyond the scope of practice for a chiropractic doctor, but what happens to the patient after the surgery?

That is essentially what this section discusses. For example, in the case of a whiplash where the patient has hit his or her head on the dashboard of the car, there will be direct trauma to the head; additionally, there will usually be trauma to the neck as well.

A person may get hit in the head with a baseball or football and sustain damage to the head, but the neck may also be damaged. In order to care for the patient properly, the doctor must look for obvious damage. As many changes in the body may take place later, it is necessary to look a little further down the road.

Recently I was told about a patient of a chiropractor who had been hit by a car while she was a pedestrian. She had hit her head on the ground, been rendered unconscious, taken to the hospital and operated on for bleeding in the head. Subsequent to her injuries, she started having seizures and, although she had never had a history of epilepsy, she was then diagnosed as an epileptic. Since medication did not control the seizures, the parents eventually took her to see a chiropractor.

After a careful analysis, the chiropractor made a determination that her atlas (C1) had been rotated out of its normal position and was putting pressure on the brain stem. This was due to the force of the impact and the resulting blow to the head. He began adjusting her atlas, very gently at first, and the seizures began to diminish. After a few months, they stopped altogether.

This case demonstrates the need for chiropractic and medicine to work together in many instances. The chiropractor could not have performed the operation that saved the girl's life, and the surgeon could never have moved the atlas back into its proper position to stop the seizures.

There are many other symptoms which may be the result of a blow to the head. These include dizziness, nausea, blindness, deafness, an inability to smell or taste, a loss of memory, narcolepsy (excessive sleep), and a decrease in the overall immune system; causing frequent colds, flus, and allergies.

Many times these symptoms can be traced to the area of the brain which has been damaged. Often these may go undetected because chiropractors are usually the only ones who can detect cervical or neck misalignment. This is especially true when you, the family member, may be told by the medical doctor that they can't find anything wrong with your loved one. The only thing they are able to do is give drugs to decrease the symptoms.

If you do take them to see a chiropractor and the chiropractor is able to help, then get the M.D. and the D.C. together to discuss the case and the contribution each of them has made. This might prevent needless suffering of future patients who might be helped by a combined effort of these two disciplines. It would certainly contribute to the understanding each may have of the other's science.

4

Other Joints of the Body—
Why They Hurt?

If you walk, your feet are your foundation.

Many people are surprised to hear that chiropractors work on areas of the body other than the spine. When you think about the spine, it is simply a series of joints which function best when aligned properly. It is the same with the other joints of the body.

Shoulder Pain

In this section we are discussing pain that is related strictly to the shoulder, as in direct trauma. This section is not about disorders which come from the neck. It has become increasingly popular for people in their 30's and 40's to return to the sports of their childhood, such as weekend and evening games of softball, touch football (even tackle!), and other contests in which great demands are placed on the shoulder. Consequently, chiropractors are seeing a big increase in shoulder problems.

The shoulder does not bear any weight like the hips and knees, nor does it have to accommodate for different types of running surfaces like the feet do. However, from an engineering standpoint, it is one of the worst constructed joints of the body. There are no bony attachments, and it is held together entirely by soft tissues such as ligaments, tendons and muscles.

As such, it is subject to all of the problems we have discussed regarding damage to soft tissues. We see a variety of strains, sprains, tears, dislocations and in general, a buildup of scar tissue over the years as the joint is repeatedly damaged and the healing process continues.

Often a patient will present a shoulder problem which is aggravated by use. In exploring the history, you find that he or she

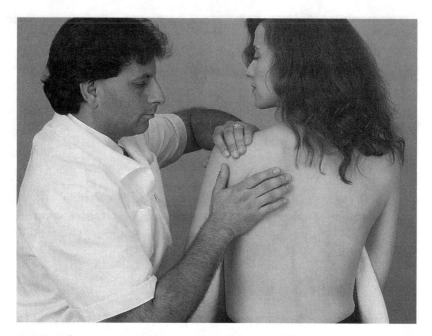

Here the chiropractor checks and adjusts the shoulder of a patient.

has worked very hard at an occupation which demands a great deal of hand, arm or shoulder motion. If x-rays are taken, they can show that there has actually been bone added to the shoulder joint. This is because other areas of the soft tissue have eroded away. In effect, the joint has simply worn out.

If this is the case and there is extra bone growth, it may have to be removed surgically. Before surgery, the surgeon or chiropractor will probably order an MRI or CAT scan to verify the extent of the damage to the shoulder. If and when surgery is done, the doctor may do a simple arthroscopy (small incision and view with a scope) and if needed, more extensive work will be performed.

My good friend Dale, who fine tunes and rebuilds racing motorcycles, recently had to have shoulder surgery. After extensive diagnostic tests his surgeon informed him that his shoulder was simply "worn out." His pain was increasing, he was getting weaker and was rapidly losing range of motion. He did the smart thing, though. He tried conservative chiropractic care first, which helped, but not enough. Then he tried medication. Finally, surgery was the only option remaining. He is post-surgical now and doing much

better, but is still under chiropractic care because the nerves leading into his shoulder are slightly compressed as they exit the neck.
Cervical adjusting helps to decrease the pressure on the nerves.

Often we get patients who say the problem with their shoulder is that it keeps dislocating when they do a certain motion. It
actually rolls out of its socket, either by accident or on purpose;
some people can force the shoulder to dislocate (such as Mel
Gibson in "Lethal Weapon II"). One thing to consider is that
chiropractors are specially trained at stretching out tight, fibrotic
tissues. That's our job—to stretch the soft tissue and remove the
nerve interference so the body can heal itself.

However, if the joint has been stretched over and over, we are
limited in what we can do. Sometimes setting the joint and
specialized taping for several months can help, as taught by Kevin
Hearon, D.C., C.C.S.P. If there is too much damage, the services
of a surgeon who specializes in shoulder repair might be required.

Suppose you have been throwing a baseball since you were a
little kid, then in high school you discovered the joys of love and
kind of lost interest in getting sweaty, dusty and dirty on the field.
Now, you are a little older and are rediscovering the fun of throwing a baseball or football—or any sport which requires movement
of your shoulder. You may overwork it and cause pain. You may
move the long bone of the arm (humerus) slightly out of its normal
position, causing a constant rub and strain. Or you may tear part of
the bursa (fluid-filled sac surrounding the joint), and scar tissue
starts to form. If it inflames due to trauma or overuse, bursitis
develops.

The chiropractor will analyze the shoulder, diagnose the
problem, and reset the shoulder properly in its natural position
and/or work out the adhesive scar tissue. It is also advantageous to
do trigger point therapy, which will loosen up tight, spastic
muscles. Two common areas usually worked on are the deep
bursae in the front of the shoulder joint and the muscle belly of the
infraspinatus muscle (muscle which runs from the shoulder blade
to the top of the arm).

I was interested to find an article by Donald R. Murphy, D.C. about the importance of doing infraspinatus trigger point therapy. He sees problems with the infraspinatus muscle in athletes who throw, due to the rapid deceleration after the throw is completed. Power lifters and body builders have similar troubles, due to an imbalance in the larger muscles of the chest and back and the smaller muscles of the shoulder. People with "rounded shoulders" put more strain on the infraspinatus to stabilize the head of the humerus (upper arm).[33]

The chiropractor will also analyze your neck to determine if there are any affected nerves inhibiting the body's natural tendency to heal the shoulder. If there are affected nerves or if there has been damage to any part of the shoulder, some healing time will be required. If the nerves exiting the neck are impinged in any way, there will probably be a slower recovery time.

Arms and Hands

Any time the extremities such as legs, feet, arms and hands hurt, the chiropractor is faced with a challenge. Many things can cause this type of pain, including the spine. In medicine, the primary concern is the symptoms and the doctor might only look at the extremity in question and may ignore any spinal involvement. Unfortunately, sometimes medicine is primarily a fix-the-symptom-as-you-go type of therapy.

Chiropractors usually think in terms of fixing the source of the problem and, for the most part, ignoring the symptoms. This may sound strange, but it allows us to get to the heart of the matter. If there is pain somewhere in the arm or the hand, the chiropractor should check all the way back to the neck where the nerves exit and above, up to the very top vertebrae of the neck. If a problem exists, the chiropractor will want to work on the neck because he or she knows the recuperative powers of the body will be enhanced if the neck is cleared of subluxations. All the healing power of the body comes from the brain, and if there is any blockage of this communication, there will be a reduced degree of healing. Our job is to remove nerve interference wherever it exists, so the body can do what it was designed to do—heal itself.

One analogy for the nervous system could be a wiring system which goes from the brain (power company) to your hands (the lights in your house) in a two-way connection. The brain also serves as the meter reader, determining not just how much power is used, but also how much is needed at all times. As with any power failure, the problem may be at the plant (brain), in the wires to the house (spinal cord), in the house (shoulder and arms), or in the light bulb (wrist and arms).

It could be that there is something wrong in both the wrist and the neck, in which case the chiropractor would treat both. This is especially likely in the case of people who use their hands constantly and also hold their shoulders in a shrugged position, such as surgeons, nurses, hair stylists, barbers, computer users, professional drivers, or commuters. Tension is created in the shoulders which causes the nerves coming out of the neck to compress. This could cause pain there as well as down the arms. Any time a nerve is damaged, dysfunction may occur anywhere along its course. This is why chiropractors are very successful with these types of conditions. Our approach incorporates the body as a whole, not just a collection of independent parts.

Elbow

Most of us have knocked our elbows on some hard surface which sends instant and temporary tingling down into the hand. We call this hitting our funny bone, but there is usually nothing funny about it—it hurts! The elbow is a relatively simple joint made up of three bones: humerus above and radius and ulna below. Usually it is the ulna or inside bone which is the one that is involved. This is because the corresponding nerve is the ulnar nerve which passes through the elbow on the inside and goes into the little finger and part of the ring finger.

Problems may occur if there has been damage to the bony structure of the elbow. The bones rarely dislocate as with the shoulder, but they may subluxate. This can make you feel like you are constantly hitting your "funny bone," even when you are not. It is very common for chiropractors to adjust the elbow. Usually it is the radius which moves out of position, but the ulna also subluxates.

One patient in our clinic came to see us with a post-surgical elbow which gave her a great deal of trouble. She had injured it at work by doing repetitive motions as an receptionist/office clerk. The surgeon did a good job of removing the scar tissue around the nerve and releasing the joint, but when the operation was over her ulna and radius were both out of position. She had had extensive post-surgical physical therapy, exercise, and even an MRI scan, but no one could help her.

After adjusting the elbow and applying some microcurrent physical therapy, she recovered almost 100% of her pre injury range-of-motion with no more pain. This not only made us look good, but it made the surgeon look good. When she came in for care, she was sure he had messed up her elbow for life and was very unhappy. This is one more example where chiropractic can be a valuable adjunct to medical care.

Hands

There are several reasons why your hands may hurt. It could be that there is pain radiating down your entire arm. Understand, that it may be one or both arms. As discussed previously, a cervical disc protrusion or pressure on the nerve from a misaligned vertebra or a pinched nerve could cause the symptom. It could be that the bones in the hands (carpal bones) have misaligned and are pinching the nerves. It could also be that the tendons or ligaments in the hands have become inflamed and are hurting. It could be one of the many arthritises, such as rheumatoid or degenerative. It might also be carpal tunnel syndrome where the nerves leading into the palm of the hand have become entrapped, due to chronic pressure by the soft tissues of the hand. This occurs with overuse of the hand and can be very debilitating. The bones of the hands can be adjusted back into their normal position just as the bones of the arm. If there is scar tissue putting pressure on the nerves, adjusting the hands may stretch the scar tissue and realign the bones away from the nerves.

Carpal Tunnel Syndrome

No chapter on the disorders of the hands would be complete without some discussion of carpal tunnel syndrome. This has become the hot topic among patients, doctors, therapists and insurance companies. It may be characterized as numbness or tingling in the wrists and hands. There may be weakness of the hands and an inability to hold certain objects. The symptoms may get worse after long periods of using the hands or wrists.

Some actions which may cause carpal tunnel syndrome are typing, giving injections, using a screwdriver, knitting, or any activity which causes the hands to be extended backwards or at a poor angle for continuous periods of time. As the patient uses the wrists over and over, inflammation may build up. If it occurs in the tendons, we know it as tendonitis. When this occurs repeatedly, scar tissue may build up in the wrists, and the patient feels chronic pain at the site of the injury.

The nerve which moves through the carpal bones of the wrist may become trapped and squeezed. Kevin Hearon, D.C., C.C.S.P., a Certified Chiropractic Sports Physician, has proposed that the problem be called "carpal flat syndrome" because the mechanism of injury is usually with the hands arched up, causing the carpal bones to flatten out and compress the nerves.

The symptoms may be controlled and possibly corrected with chiropractic adjusting of the carpal bones of the hand, as mentioned above. In actuality, Dr. Hearon has remarkable success with his patients by adjusting the offending carpal bone off the nerve and then taping the hand into the corrective position. He then shows the patient how to tape up their own hand and wrist. He says that after three months of being taped in the corrected position, the ligaments will restructure themselves accordingly. This could open up the canals through which the nerves pass and help keep them open.

The chiropractor may also use microcurrent or ultrasound therapy on the inflamed tissue. However, if there is too much scar tissue, surgery may be inevitable. Sometimes a chiropractor and a medical doctor will work together on these types of cases, combining both sciences. They would likely combine adjusting, physical therapy, anti-inflammatory drugs, and painkillers. This may be the best answer for carpal tunnel patients who have extensive damage.

Of course, you want the cause of the problem to be corrected, so the inflammation doesn't recur. If the set-up of your job station causes continued problems, your chiropractor may go to your office and make ergonomic changes, if he or she has been trained to do that. There will be more on this in the chapter on insurance.

Hips

The hips are the joints of the body which connect the legs to the pelvis and the rest of the spine. There are many things which can go wrong with these weight-bearing joints. It is important to realize that the hips can be adjusted if they are out of their normal position, just like the other joints of the body could be adjusted.

The hip is put together as a "ball and socket" type of joint. The ball is the head of the femur, which is the long bone of the leg. The socket is on the side of the pelvis and holds the femur head. The femur may become jammed into the socket, displaced either forward or backwards, and over time wear down the soft tissues which surround the joint. It is rare for the femur to become completely displaced like the shoulder because of the extreme stability created by the "ball and socket" configuration.

The hip can be the site of painful arthritises such as rheumatoid and degenerative. The hip may have a congenital problem such as hip dysplasia (see "Anomalies" in Appendix B) or become fractured in a fall. If this occurs, there may be damage to the femur, the acetabulum, or both. Osteoporosis may develop and cause the femur head actually to protrude through the acetabulum in a condition known as "acetabuli protrosio," caused by the weight of the body. Indeed, this may occur as a result of many different types of bone diseases.

Chiropractic care in the hip region is limited to increasing ranges of motion and attempting to "reset the joint" into its proper

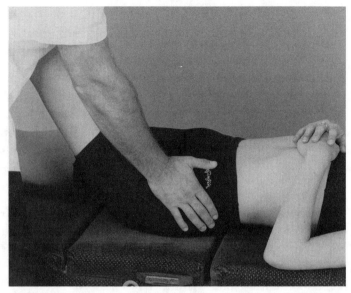

Here the chiropractor is setting the left hip into it's proper position.

anatomical position by manipulation. However, a chiropractic adjustment adds benefit to almost any condition if a subluxation exists in the region of the spine where there is a neurological connection to the hip area. If a subluxation exists at the spinal level corresponding to the hip, there will be a decrease in healing potential of the area and, in fact, the healing will take much longer.

Knees

Knee problems can be frustrating for both the patient and the practitioner. The knees support the weight of almost the entire body. They are constantly demanded to bend, twist, turn, and support weight. They are subject to great compressive forces and incredible amounts of torque.

For example, let's take the golf swing. The knees have to support the weight of the golfer, turn in different directions, and torque to a high degree of strain. On the beginning of the downswing, one knee drives into the ball while the other stays torqued and straight. Finally, both knees move forward together and end up with the opposite one torqued and straight. Just imagine the stress on your knees during your favorite exercise or sport!

The knee is set up as a hinged joint, made up of the tibial plateau (lower leg) with condyles below and the femoral (upper leg or thigh) condyles above. Between them is a disc pad known as the meniscus. Holding these joints together are the cruciate ligaments inside and the patellar, collateral and fibular head ligaments on the outside. In addition, there are a multitude of tendons and muscles holding the joint together. Overlaying the whole joint is the patella or knee cap.

The knees are subject to the arthritises mentioned above. In addition to a direct trauma, such as a football injury, indirect trauma, such ankle or hip problems, or bad posture can cause abnormal stresses. One of the interesting features of a knee injury is that it may not hurt until the next day.

What often causes the most pain is not the damage to the body part, but the resultant swelling which occurs as the body tries to fix the problem on its own. As you continue to walk (or limp) around, your body weight is compressing the knee together, keeping much of the fluid out. When you lay down at night, all of the weight is off and the knee is free to swell its heart out. In the morning if you can't get out of bed, your first reaction is, "What the heck did I do?"

If the blow or trauma to the knee was minor, patients under my care go home and use the R.I.C.E. formula: rest, ice, compression, and elevation (of the leg). If the trauma was serious or they just want to be sure, they might come in for an evaluation and treatment. If you are injured and see an M.D., remember that he or she may just look at the knee and not bother to check your spine. You may have had one or more vertebrae subluxated in your lower back, which will have to be reset before complete healing of the knee can occur.

As mentioned above, if your posture is abnormal, all the joints on one side of your body will have to work harder to compensate. This may include both knees. Just ask yourself this question: How important to me is walking?

The chiropractor will conduct a careful analysis of your knee and decide if it is a chiropractic problem or if it needs to be handled medically. The chiropractor can increase the range of motion in the joint and, as with the hip, may actually adjust the knee.

For example, if the leg or thigh has become twisted or torqued, the chiropractor may gently distract the leg, torque in the opposite direction, and reset the joint. Someone else or the patient may stabilize the thigh in order to isolate the knee joint. This technique is taught by Abby Irwin, D.C., C.C.S.P. of Oakland, California who works with hundreds of athletes every year. She was a longtime associate of Jan Corwin, D.C., C.C.S.P. one of the U.S. Olympic Team chiropractors.

If the knee has simply become compressed, the chiropractor may use simple distraction (traction) methods to relieve the area. If the knee has rotated or become torqued, then the chiropractor may use Harrison Biophysics, Activator Method or a distraction combined with a slight rotation method. However, as with the

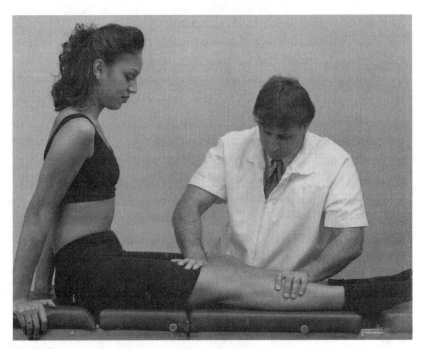

The chiropractic knee adjustment on a drop table.

hip example above, there are areas of the spine which correspond to the knee joint. If these areas are subluxated, the chances of the knee ever healing completely while compression on the nerve exists is unlikely. This is why a chiropractor should be consulted whenever a problem exists in one of the extremities.

One patient of mine is a marathon runner who runs 60 to 80 miles per week. He came in with pain on the outside of his knee and tingling in his foot. He was misdiagnosed for over a year, and his mileage dropped to 20 miles per week. With one adjustment to his fibula (outside bone of the leg) the pain and tingling stopped immediately. The original trauma to the knee was actually a twisted ankle. He is now back to his long distance running.

Ankles and Feet

The ankles and feet are the last joints of the extremities we will be examining. It's true that you can have the healthiest spine in the world, but if your feet or ankles are unbalanced, you may be subject to back problems.

An easy check you can do regarding your feet is to look at the way your shoes wear down. Do the outside of the heels wear down first or the insides? Is there a tremendous amount of wear on one part of your shoes or is the wear evenly distributed throughout? Have your chiropractor look at your shoes and ask if this could be contributing to your spinal problems.

Kevin Hearon, D.C., C.C.S.P., carefully examines the wear on the shoe and also the areas of the feet which are calloused and worn. Then he can diagnose abnormal walking and the resulting compensating patterns. From this information he can often predict future foot, spine and health problems.

Despite the fact that the ankles support the entire weight of the body, they are one of the weakest joints and the most prone to repeated injury in the entire body. How many people do you know who continuously sprain an ankle over and over again? As the ligaments weaken and stretch they become more unstable and will be even more likely to sprain again in the future.

This may require an entire program of care, including adjusting the back, the ankle, and feet (by the chiropractor), stretching some muscles, tendons, and ligaments, and strengthening others, along with repetition of prescribed exercises.

The feet and ankles may need to be taped in order to stabilize them. Finally, orthotics that are cast to form a corrective moulding of the feet may need to be prescribed. You and the chiropractor may even consult with a podiatrist or orthopedist to see if a medical problem exists.

One reason the outside of the ankle sprains more easily (inversion sprain) than the inside of the ankle (eversion sprain) is the difference in the ankle's anatomy. On the inside of the ankle is the tough deltoid ligament which resists stretching of any kind, while on the outside of the ankle is the somewhat weaker talofibular ligament which is much more prone to sprain.

My patient R was playing basketball a few years ago on a court which was about 4 inches higher than the surrounding

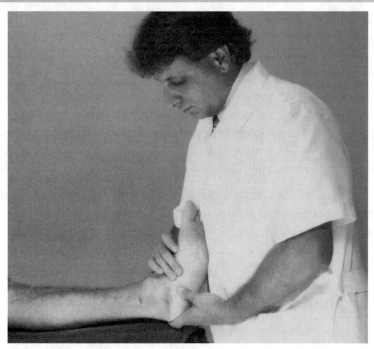

Here the chiropractor checks and adjusts a badly sprained ankle.

asphalt. R came down with a rebound (he's 6'7") and slipped his right foot slightly off the court. This caused an eversion sprain as the deltoid ligament blew out. Being the dynamic and athletic individual he is, R spun around and caused an inversion sprain of the same foot as the talofibular ligament broke. He said he heard two loud "pops" and that was the end of his basketball and running activities for the next 2 ½ years.

When R came to me at the student clinic at Life Chiropractic College West in San Lorenzo, California, I began a program of care designed to realign his feet, ankles (the left one had carried most of the weight from the time of the accident), knees, hips, and spine. As a result of this accident, painful scar tissue had been allowed to form which caused him to walk unevenly. Eventually, with adjustments and ultrasound on the ankle to break up the scar tissue, he was able to regain his normal walk and to run and play basketball again.

To give you an idea of how health deteriorates and is regained in cycles, because of his lack of exercise R had gained weight which put an even greater stress on his legs and back. Once he began to regain his health, he exercised and lost the excess weight. With the weight off, there was less stress on the joints and he began to improve even faster.

There are so many problems with the feet that an entire profession dedicated solely (no pun intended!) to them has developed. These doctors are known as podiatrists, and although their school curriculum is closely related to medical doctors and chiropractors, they are experts on the feet and only treat the feet.

What a chiropractor may offer you in the way of foot care is limited to realignment of misaligned bones or joints of the feet, taping, and orthotics. Just as with the hands, the feet are made up of several small bones called tarsal bones. These may become misaligned just as the spine might misalign and may cause pain and problems with walking. The chiropractor is trained to gently adjust the feet back into their normal position.

If the problem persists a consultation with a podiatrist or an orthopedist may be needed. The rule in my office is that if I can't give the patient considerable relief in four or five adjustments, then I send them downstairs to the podiatrist, Dr. Jonathan Steinberg. Usually, if a patient hasn't responded to my treatments, Dr. Steinberg will find something extensively wrong, and I can rest assured the problem is being resolved.

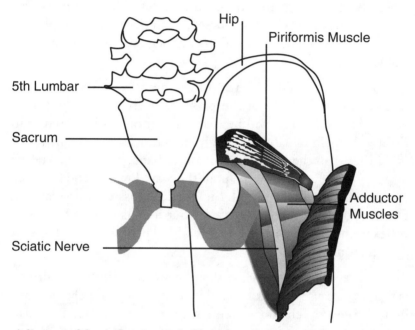

A diagram of the piriformis muscle. Notice how the piriformis lays over the sciatic nerve. It may compress the nerve against the adductor muscles.

Piriformis Syndrome — Sciatica & Pelvic Pain

Piriformis syndrome is one of the most overlooked problems a patient can present. The piriformis muscle originates at the side of the tailbone or sacrum and stretches over to the head of the femur. This is where the sciatic nerve exits the pelvic region. All of the muscles which work to pull your leg closer to the midline of your body (called adductors) lie under this nerve with the exception of the piriformis muscle.

As you might expect, this muscle, when pulled tight enough, will press onto the sciatic nerve and cause pain to radiate down the leg. This is also known as "peripheral nerve entrapment syndrome," because the sciatic nerve is the peripheral nerve and the piriformis muscle is entrapping it. Piriformis muscle spasm is extremely painful and often difficult to diagnose. Here the old saying applies, "If you never look, you won't find it!"

In some cases the sciatic nerve actually pierces the piriformis muscle and may become stretched and deformed as the muscle itself stretches and becomes adhered. As in the above example, the pain may radiate down the back of the leg and may also develop paresthesias (tingling).[34]

Piriformis Syndrome will often mimic a lumbar vertebral disc syndrome because of the pressure it creates on the sciatic nerve. The difference will be that if the problem is muscular in nature, the pain radiating through the buttocks will usually travel no farther than the knees. On the other hand, a lumbar vertebral disc syndrome may cause pain all the way down to the foot and could cause muscular atrophy in the leg (loss of musculature), foot drop (where you cannot raise your foot as you walk), loss of reflexes in the leg, bowel and bladder problems, and sexual dysfunction.

Another interesting clinical finding with piriformis syndrome is that it can cause different areas in the front of your pelvis to hurt. This is seen much more frequently in women, but it is also observed in men. The pain may mimic things such as ovarian cysts, salpingitis (inflammation of the fallopian tubes), sexually transmitted diseases which cause pain, vaginal spasms, hernias, or bladder infection. There have even been cases of impotency in men and painful intercourse in women.

The difficulty here is trying to tell the difference between pain in an organ that is caused by a problem in that organ and pain being referred from constriction on the sciatic nerve, due to pressure from the piriformis muscle. To go one step further, does the pressure on the sciatic nerve cause pain and disease in the region of the pelvic bowl? Before you decide to have surgery for pelvic pain of an unknown origin, have someone who is qualified evaluate your piriformis muscle for a potential problem. Usually a diagnosis can be made by pressing on the piriformis muscle or by stretching it to see if this produces pain.

Patients are always asking me what causes piriformis syndrome. Well, actually they ask me, "Why does my butt hurt?" One of the major causes is having a wallet in your back pocket for many years while sitting or driving. This causes direct pressure on the muscle and the nerve. Overuse of the piriformis is also a cause and is seen in people such as long distance runners or people who don't stretch out properly before exercising.

All of these reasons cause the piriformis muscle to form microtears, resulting in the formation of scar tissue. This causes constriction and adhesions. Disruption of the proper blood flow to the muscle will cause necrosis, or death of the tissue. This in turn causes more pain. There are some very good piriformis stretches demonstrated in the exercise section of the book.

5

Subluxation and Bad Health—
The Connection

The power that made the body is the power that heals the body.

— A chiropractic tenet.

The Famous "Pinched Nerve" Theory

Chiropractors try to talk to their patients about their health, and patients want to talk to their chiropractors about their pain. Even though these two subjects may seem to be unrelated, there is a connection. As mentioned previously, the subluxation is what chiropractors are trying to correct. Subluxations are often painful, but not always so. Subluxations usually cause problems with a person's health; however, this connection is often not made.

The purpose of this chapter is to show how chiropractic, through its unique approach to health, has some benefit to the many problems which plague mankind. Understand also that the purpose of this book is to simplify your understanding of what chiropractors do.

Unfortunately, neurology is very complicated. When I talk about a pinched nerve, it is important for you to know that it is really a sensory nerve reaction reflex loop that has gone haywire. The sensory nerve has detected a problem and has communicated and commanded a bodily response; however, the response may be too strong for the situation.

There are three main causes of these adverse reflex nerve reaction loops:

1. ***The vertebral or bone-out-of-place model:*** This model has been used by chiropractors for the last 100 years, and by European bone setters and Egyptians for thousands of years. What happens

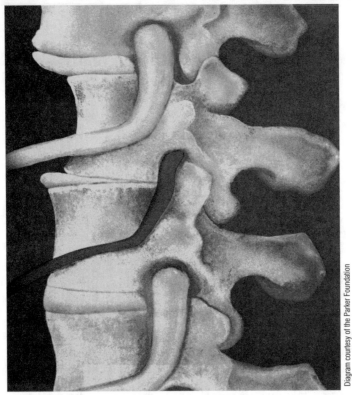

Diagram courtesy of the Parker Foundation

The diagram shows a "pinched" nerve exiting the spine. Notice how this nerve has atrophied and appears diseased? Also notice how the vertebrae has pushed backwards into the spinal canal.

is that one or more vertebrae move out of position with respect to the vertebrae above and below. The movement is usually very slight, but enough to cause swelling in the soft tissues surrounding the joint. This "malposition," if you will, puts pressure on one or more of the nerves as they exit the spine.

Some chiropractors view the spine as more a dynamic structure in constant motion rather than a stack of bones. These doctors prefer to view subluxations as restrictions in motion, like a stuck hinge on a gate, rather than a vertebra out of place—like one stone pushed out in an otherwise smooth rock wall. This is why the terms "vertebrae out of place" and "pinched nerves" give rise to new definitions as we learn more about the spine.

For convenience and tradition, definitions are sometimes mentioned and used in this book. One of the newest definitions as stated by Daniel Murphy, D.C., D.A.B.C.O., is that a subluxation is "a mechanical lesion that creates chronic sensory bed disturbance causing reflexes that alter the function of the efferent nervous system causing muscular and visceral dysfunction." In effect, this means that when vertebrae misalign, they create a reflex which changes muscle tone and organ function (in a bad way). In fact, muscle spasm, organ disease and even degenerated discs themselves cause feedback which makes the subluxated vertebrae worse. Essentially, you have a catch–22 situation. This loop cannot be broken by itself. It can be changed only by a chiropractic adjustment.

The spine is the structure which holds the nerves as they travel from the brain to every organ, gland, muscle, and tissue of the body and back again. The nerves run through the spinal column and also out each side at each level. If a vertebra has shifted its position, the swelling created could actually contact or "pinch" the nerve. The pain you feel may be of a sharp pinching nature, or it may be dull and achy if it has been there for a long time.

The nerves that bring sensation messages from the body to the spine (afferent) go in the back of the vertebrae, the posterior horn cells, and up to the brain. The responding signal is then sent from the brain down the spine and out at the same spinal level. The motor nerve exits the front of the spinal cord (efferent), through the anterior horn cells, and carries the message (the brain's response to the sensation) back out to the rest of the body. There is a split in this nerve; one branch goes to the muscles and is called the motor efferent and the other branch goes to all of the organs in the body and is called the preganglionic sympathetic efferents.

Depending on where or which nerve is "pinched," or better yet "stimulated," you would experience different or possibly no symptoms at all. As the nerve is stimulated to react to the detected problem, it will not shut down, but will fire faster and faster. If the nerve is "pinched," you might feel weakness in the area the nerve leads to or you may experience a change in sensation such as numbness, tingling, heaviness, pain or hypersensitivity. You might even feel as though you have little ants crawling on that area of your body (paresthesias).

Lastly, if the nerve leading to the sympathetic ganglion chain is affected, you may experience no pain at all, but may be heading for an early grave if the organs of the body at the end of the nerves lose their function and begin to die off. Should this happen, the organs to that corresponding area would be weaker and become subject to invasion by different bacteria which normally are at peace with the body, or attacked by a circulating virus. The essence of this is that you would probably get sick. Your own functioning immune system would go to work, but it may be too late.[35]

If you continue to let it go, you would probably need to see an M.D. for drugs and/or possible surgery. Even if the medicine or surgery is "successful," you are still treating results, not causes. Isn't it better to take 45 minutes to get checked out by a good chiropractor? Nowhere is the old adage "an ounce of prevention is worth a pound of cure" more applicable than in chiropractic care. This ounce of prevention can, has, and will save lives and decrease suffering.

2.   *Posture abnormalities:* A second way the organs and body can be affected is by postural abnormalities. We have already discussed why posture is important in the realm of back pain. Now we will explore why posture is a major contributor to systemic health.

Recall that in previous chapters, we discussed how important it is for oxygen to reach the organs and tissues of the body via the blood supply in order for a person to be healthy. Thus, anything which may deprive or reduce oxygen and nutrients from getting to the tissues will perpetuate disease, degeneration, and possibly lead to premature death. According to Irvin Korr, Ph.D., when you control the blood supply to a given area, you control tissue life, capacity to recover, resist infection, survive and maintain its integrity as a tissue.[36]

The sympathetic nervous system, as it exits from the spinal cord, controls the amount of blood which reaches the organs and tissues of the body supplied by that region of the spine. In the vertebrae-out-of-place theory that we spoke of previously, abnormal posture will cause your weight-bearing ability to be off-center, and the pressure around the nerves will increase.

Recall the work cited by Alf Brieg, M.D. (note 16–Ch.3, p. 53) which showed that abnormal posture caused changes in the spinal cord. The tiny nerves became stretched and began to bleed internally. This led to damage to the spinal nerves as they exited the spine; disease was the eventual result. Both of these conditions cause the classic "subluxations" chiropractors correct and or resolve.

The additional problems due to postural changes are found in the Korr papers where Dr. Korr makes the distinction that musculoskeletal dysfunctions around the weight-bearing parts of the axial skeleton cause pain and sustained nervous system sympathetic overload (sympathicotonia). This means that when your posture is bad, you set yourself up for continuous visceral (internal organ) dysfunction and disease due to improper shifts in the blood flow.

In 1957, Freeman concluded that shifts in gravity (postural misalignments) in the aging population led to hemorrhoids, varicose veins of the legs, osteoporosis, intestinal problems, overall poorer health and even early death.[37]

John Lennon, et. al., in 1994 concluded that posture affects all human function including proper breathing, musculoskeletal pain, mind/body interaction and balance, vocal ability—including speaking and singing, proper immune function and, of course, overall health.[38]

Normal sympathetic tone (spine free of subluxations) keeps the blood vessels open to approximately half their maximum diameter, which is normal. This helps to regulate the proper amount of blood being delivered to the visceral organs.

Picture the caveman peacefully munching his dinner of greens and animal meat. The organs are working to digest his meal and most of the blood is going to the abdominal organs. He is under parasympathetic tone and is relaxing. Suddenly a predator appears and wants to make the caveman his dinner! He jumps up and begins to run. Now he is under the same sort of sympathetic stimulation as in a subluxation, but to a much higher degree. The sympathetic nervous system has taken over, diverted most of his blood into the skeletal muscles (so he can jump away and run) and away from the digestive organs. The brain knows it can return to digest the food later, but right now it does not want to become food!

As the subluxation continues, the sympathetic nervous system nerves will fire over and over very rapidly. This is called "denervation supersensitivity" and causes the blood vessels at the end of the nerves to constrict, or become smaller. This obviously results in less blood and oxygen being delivered to that area; sickness and disease can result because lack of oxygen is the basis of cell disease and degeneration.

Most blood vessels constrict by sympathetic stimulation; the most susceptible ones are those of the abdominal viscera and the skin of the limbs. The medullary hormones, such as epinephrine and norepinephrine, are released by the adrenal medullae under sympathetic stimulation. This causes an even greater degree of blood vessel constriction which occurs at the same time of sympathetic stimulation.

A loss of blood to an area causes it to be more susceptible to viral and bacterial invasions, as well as toxins, and less able to recover from such infections.[39] The longer the condition manifests itself, the more damage will result. This is important when evaluating how chronic the problem is and trying to determine what the actual event was which caused the disease in the first place. Much of this is discussed by Dr. James M. Allen in the *Chiropractic Journal of Australia*.[40]

The chiropractor will work on your posture and begin to change it back to its ideal structure. As this occurs the nerves will resume their normal position and the denervation supersensitivity should diminish. The result is that the blood vessels will dilate and begin to deliver the proper amount of blood to the areas in question. This leads to normal tissue health and normal functioning of the body. It is this concept which supports the opening premise that chiropractors do not heal, only the body heals.[41]

3.   *Upper cervical nerve pressure:* The third way the organs are affected by the nerves is by upper cervical nerve pressure, direct pressure on the brain stem as it exits the skull. The brain and the spinal cord, the central nervous system, are responsible for 100% of the functioning of the body. Different parts of the brain are responsible for different functions.

The cerebral hemisphere controls higher thoughts, sensation and fine motor control of the body. The cerebellum coordinates all movements of the body; the body would not be able to perform even the simplest function, were it not for the cerebellum's coordinating efforts.

Then there is the brain stem which is located below the cerebellum. The brain stem contains the exit points for the cranial nerves. These control smell, sight, taste, facial sensation, facial movement, hearing, balance, shoulder movement, swallowing and tongue movement. The centers that control breathing and respiration are also on the brain stem.

As long as the brain stem is centered where it exits the skull, then passes uninterrupted through the top two vertebrae (atlas and axis), everything is okay. The problem occurs when the atlas (C1) or axis (C2) shift to one side or the other. This causes a compressive force on the brain stem which may adversely affect the nerves all the way down the body. Specifically, it could cause problems as diverse as headaches, loss of coordination, breathing difficulties, Sudden Infant Death Syndrome (SIDS) and others.

Upper cervical work directly affects the central nervous system and is the exclusive realm of chiropractic. This is where "chiropractic miracles" occur, such as helping diabetes, improving mental disorders, stabilizing blood pressure, eliminating allergies, and a host of others. In short, any disorder of the body that includes the system organs can benefit by this type of chiropractic care.

This is the subject that some M.D.'s hate hearing us talk about, preferring to keep chiropractic in the category of Good-for-Back-Pain-Only-Doctors. In most cases we are not treating those diseases as much as we are treating the back for subluxations and disorders. It's just that the nerves of the spine are attached to the organs via the autonomic nervous system, and people often get well if their back is adjusted properly. Many chiropractors are now helping to either control a disease, put it into remission, or even cure it.

Some Diseases Caused by Nerve Pressure

It has often been said that chiropractors think they can cure everything, and that they should limit their attention to back pain. Chiropractors do not believe that they can cure everything. In fact, we believe we can cure nothing. We believe that the body itself can cure anything, given the right healing environment. That is all we do—provide the body with a maximum healing environment by putting the body in the right frame of mind in order for it to heal itself best.

As you read the rest of this chapter, please keep this important principle in mind: the power that made the body in most cases can heal the body. The exception is if you have let the condition go on too long, or if you continue to do the things which are killing you in the first place.

If you still doubt the healing power of chiropractic, just ask any chiropractor who has been in practice for a few years about their "miracle cases." Dr. Arlan Fuhr, the president of Activator Methods and the National Institute of Chiropractic Research, says the problem with the chiropractic profession is that we get amazing results, but we never write them down and submit them for critical review. Well, now we are starting to write them down.

1.   *Headaches:* Headaches are one of the most common and most debilitating problems health practitioners have to treat. They can also be very frustrating for both patient and doctor. More than any other malady, headaches will keep a patient moving from one form of therapy to another, and from one type of therapist to another.

A frustrated patient will usually try drugs, chiropractic adjustments, acupuncture, herbs, cold compresses, hot compresses, or anything else which comes to mind. Indeed, of the many conditions chiropractic helps, headaches consistently comprise some of our best success stories. I have many patients who have thrown away drugs, with all their bad side effects, and simply come in for an adjustment when they feel a headache coming on.

For example, there is B, a super guy who suffered from severe headaches for five years before he came to our office for care. When B was eight years old he was sleeping in a very high bunk bed. His grandfather was sleeping in the bed below. In his sleep B rolled over and fell out of the top bunk onto the floor. He was unconscious when his grandfather woke up. Thinking B had simply fallen asleep next to him, the kindly grandfather lifted him into the bottom bunk, and he climbed into the top bunk. Unfortunately, the weak bed did not support the grandfather's weight, and the top bunk bed and the grandfather crashed down on poor B!

B had been seen by top medical people who had helped his severe headaches to some degree, but never really eliminated the problem completely. His mother knew me and asked if I thought I could do anything for him. I started adjusting his back with an emphasis on his upper neck region. Within just a few days the headaches had subsided.

Then B and his family left on vacation for three weeks. Unfortunately, it was too soon to interrupt care and the headaches returned, although not as severely nor as often as before. When he returned he started care again and now rarely has any headaches at all. We adjust him at a decreasing frequency, and his adjustments are holding for longer periods of time.

We should discuss briefly the different types of the more common headaches. B's headache might be known as a trauma-induced headache. A fairly complete description of the different types of headaches can be found in the *Merck Manual*. However, you should be cautioned that neither this book, or any other book can give you a true diagnosis of your problem. Only a qualified chiropractor or medical doctor can do that, and you should seek his or her advice on your problem as soon as possible.

Migraine: Migraines are quite common and are usually characterized as a pounding, throbbing vascular type of headache. A patient may or may not experience an "aurora" or a visual disturbance prior to an attack. There may be sensitivity to light, nausea and/or vomiting. The pain usually begins at the eyes and spreads to either or both sides of the head.

There are many presumed causes of migraines. Vascular problems, family history of the disease, diet, blood pressure, stress, and last, but certainly not least, subluxated vertebrae in the neck or cervical region can all lead to migraines. In our office and in many of my colleagues' offices, we have been able to help patients when many other systems of health care have failed by affecting the subluxated vertebrae and repositioning the bones back into their normal position.

The cervical region of the spinal cord is different from the rest of the spine in one very important respect. There is an artery called the vertebral artery which carries a great amount of blood to the brain from the heart. It passes on a (hopefully) straight course on each side of each vertebra through the transverse processes, and forms, along with the carotid arteries, the basis of the main source of the blood that goes throughout the brain.

A migraine is caused by changes in the amount of blood flow to the brain. Usually the flow decreases for some reason and then the body overcompensates by sending too much blood to the brain. The result is a pounding, vascular headache.

When vertebrae are misaligned in the neck, the vertebral artery, instead of passing straight through the vertebrae, becomes twisted and torqued. It is difficult for the blood to flow straight and evenly to the brain. When a chiropractor aligns the vertebrae, the result is a much more even flow of blood.

Another method for treating migraines is to apply microamperage current to the suboccipital muscle. Microamperage is distinguished from units such as TENS units, as they are in the milliamperage range, which is 1,000 times more powerful than micro units such as the Myomatic. The Myomatic actually recreates the body's own natural healing frequencies, so it is essentially the same as the body. The only difference is that the healing time is greatly reduced.

The Myomatic has become famous in athletic circles for being the treatment of choice for injuries. Athletes such as Jerry Rice and Joe Montana of the San Francisco 49ers, Olympic stars such as Carl Lewis, Jackie Joyner-Kersey and Ben Johnson, Warriors and Lakers basketball team members, and many others have all benefitted from this therapy. Many athletes now own their own machines.

Tension Headaches: Tension headaches are some of the most common headaches to plague men and women. What causes tension headaches? TENSION!! It's no wonder this happens, given the life most of us lead. We are always trying to cram 20 hours of work into an eight-hour day. Even when we are supposed to be resting, we find ways to add stress and tension to our lives.

There is an important lesson here for all of us. A few years ago I took a seminar with Dan Millman, the author of the best seller *The Peaceful Warrior*.[42] Dan told us that vacations were not a luxury, that they were mandatory in order to keep our sanity. I believe he is right.

Another cause of tension headaches is poor posture, especially where the head has moved forward past the shoulders or is looking downward. This is known as anterior weight bearing and has been discussed in the section on posture. Essentially what happens is that the muscles in the back of the neck are under constant stress and strain, trying to move the head back over the shoulders where it belongs.

The muscles are overworked, fatigued and begin to spasm. In turn, this constricts the blood vessels going into the scalp, causing the other muscles of the scalp to tighten and constrict. The neck vertebrae no longer function or move as they should. They may get "stuck" in certain positions.

One study found that females suffering from chronic headaches had mobility changes in their necks.[43] The classic symptoms are pain which starts at the base of the skull, moves up over the top of the head and usually lodges behind the eyes. The symptoms may be mild or rather severe. The pain may be felt on one side or both; it may even move from one side to the other. Occasionally the pain may be felt under the bones of the scalp. It might feel like a constant pressure or even a pounding sensation. Usually it is not like a vascular pounding as you might have with a migraine or other vascular headache. In some cases, one or both eyes may throb with pressure.

Care is often a combination of therapies, including cervical adjustments, muscle work on the suboccipital muscles in the back of the head, and postural adjusting to restore the natural curve to the neck and bring the head back over the shoulders. The chiropractor may loosen the region of the head at the base of the skull with deep massage for a few seconds.

Certain small nodules may be present inside the center or "belly" of the muscles of this suboccipital region. These nodules are small bundles of pain called trigger points. The chiropractor or therapist may hold these trigger points down against the scalp for at least ten seconds until they release. This is known as Trigger Point Therapy[44] and was discussed briefly in the section on shoulder injuries.

You yourself can try to massage gently or press any tight muscles in the back of your skull at the base. If it hurts a great deal or if you get no relief, stop and consult your chiropractor. You may also apply ice to the area or a cold compress for up to 20 minutes. *(See the instructions on icing in Appendix C at the end of the book.)*

The mechanism is simple. The muscles work too hard and become fatigued. By applying pressure to the muscle, the fibers are stretched beyond their present comfortable limit. This sends a message back to the spine called the stretch reflex. The golgi tendons (area of attachment on each end of the tendons) receive the message and then stretch or elongate in order to lengthen the muscle.

The practitioner and the patient usually feel the muscle bundle/trigger point relax and open. This gives a great deal of relief to the patient. However, it is important to realize that the trigger point will return if the cause of the problem is not corrected. In this case the cause would be that C1 or C2 is subluxated.

Another possible cause of pain and tension in this region is when the occiput becomes jammed into the C1 or atlas. The condyles of the atlas and the occiput stop moving freely and, just like the other joints in the spine, become swollen and put pressure on the nerves. The best care for this subluxation is an adjustment.

Sinus Headaches: Sinus headaches are usually characterized by intense pressure and/or pain in specific regions of the head, such as the forehead (frontal) or cheeks (maxillary). It is often due to the mucous which surrounds and fights the bacteria or virus of a cold while trying to destroy it. For some reason the sinus passages stop draining.

One of the problems with taking cold medications, such as antihistamines, to control the symptoms is that they inhibit the body's natural tendency to use histamine to combat the antigen that is causing the sickness. By taking these drugs you may be helping yourself feel better by reducing the swelling, but you may lengthen the duration of the cold or allergies. It is up to you to decide if you can live with the body's response to killing the "bug."

If the body's fight to cure you is making it impossible to breathe or get any rest, specific temporary drug therapy may be the best short term solution. Fever kills harmful viruses and bacteria, but if the fever gets too high in its intense fight you could die because the brain is getting overheated and blood cells and enzymes become denatured. The fever must be decreased (as an army retreats temporarily in order to regroup and reorganize) in order for you to continue to live.

Since chiropractic has historically been shown to help support and increase the efficiency of the immune system, patients often receive spinal adjustments at times when colds, allergies, and flu are on the rise. New scientific experiments by Brennan, et. al. have started the process of controlled investigation of this important relationship.[45] These researchers have shown a clear relationship between spinal adjustments and biological cellular response. Often chiropractic care is just what a patient's immune system needs in order to help it get "over the hump" in times of sickness.

In addition to adjusting the spine to help the immune system and sinuses, there is an established osteopathic technique which I use in my office. If someone has a head cold and bad sinuses, I will gently stroke my fingers down the sides of the sternocleidomastoid muscle from the head down toward the heart. The lymphatic chains located there will drain better when properly stimulated. My patient R came in with a bad head cold. After using this technique for a few minutes, he said he felt an immediate decrease of pressure in his head.

You might ask your chiropractor to try this therapy with you and also to show you how to do it on yourself. Try this in addition to other nonmedication therapies, such as heat and humidifiers you may already use.

NOTE: One important point to remember about headaches: if you have had direct trauma to the head, such as a collision, fall or auto accident, you need to be examined by a chiropractor or a medical doctor. This is also true if you have had a headache for more than a few days and there is no apparent cause, particularly if the pain continues to get worse. You may have something serious underneath, such as a broken blood vessel or a growing tumor. Don't take any chances!

2. *Asthma:* Asthma is a disease which affects millions of people each year, including a large number of children. It is characterized by shortness of breath or the inability to take a deep breath due to spasm and swelling of the small bronchi of the lungs. As they spasm, less air passes into the small sacs known as alveoli at the end of the passageways. Then the air gets trapped due to the mucous and the person cannot exhale.

A person suffering from this condition will usually have a very short intake of breath and a very long exhalation with a distinct wheezing sound. It may become so bad that the victim may experience a total inability to inhale. People have died from severe asthma attacks.

There are many things which can trigger an asthma attack. Food allergies, stress, pollens in the air and animal fur are known to elicit an asthmatic response or cause it to get worse. Even medical interventions, such as aspirin, beta-blockers and non-steroidal anti-inflammatory drugs can cause an attack.[46] In fact, some studies have shown that the dramatic rise in worldwide asthma-related death is due to medical management of asthma with beta-agonist bronchodilator inhalers.[47]

Chiropractors have known for years that asthma may be caused or worsened by pressure on the nerves in the area just below the neck, called the upper thoracics. There may exist in the upper thoracics a "dishing in," or flat spot on one or more vertebrae. Although the relationship is not yet totally clear, this pressure may affect nerves which lead to the lungs and causes the bronchi to spasm. Dr. Dean H. Lines, an Australian chiropractor, authored one study where he successfully managed three cases of asthma (two children and one adult) with a combination of chiropractic adjustments along with identifying and controlling environmental and food allergies.[48]

I have this flattening in my spine. I had asthma which never responded well to any medication, inhalation therapy or exercises. When I became a chiropractic student, Dr. Dan Murphy began adjusting my upper thoracics. He would press the ones below from back to front, creating a leverage for the ones above to move backwards. This adjustment is commonly known to chiropractors as an anterior thoracics or anterior dorsals move. The adjustment caused my spine to "open up" and allowed me to breathe freely. To this day I have never had another asthma attack, and mine used to be quite severe.

One thing we can address directly is that a person with asthma will often have a great deal of tightness in his or her back. The ribs and respiratory organs are compressed and prone to spasm. The muscles may enlarge (hypertrophy) as the person spends a lifetime fighting to breathe.

When a chiropractic adjustment is given to the spine there is a reflex relaxation which takes place and allows the ribs to move more freely. There are thousands of anecdotal cases of asthma sufferers who have responded to spinal adjustments. I have had many in my own practice.

> For example, my patient C was diagnosed as having asthma late in life. She has emphysema and other lung problems from smoking. She sustained a pre-adjustment breathing volume of fewer than 150 ml of air volume; she was literally gasping for air. After the first adjustment, her lung volume went up to over 200 ml and after the second adjustment it was over 250 ml! With support adjusting, it has continued to improve. This would merit some future study of chiropractic care for asthma sufferers. Dr. Tedd Koren cites several references for spinal adjusting to correct or help asthma in his pamphlet *"Asthma, Emphysema and Bronchitis."*[49]

3. ***Diabetes Mellitus:*** Diabetes is a fairly ancient disease which may appear in childhood or may manifest during adulthood. It is a disease where the levels of sugar (glucose) in the blood are not regulated well. When you eat a meal, the levels of sugar in the blood rise dramatically. The pancreas secretes insulin from beta cells in tissues called the islets of Langerhans. The insulin brings the sugar levels down by driving glucose into the muscular and soft tissues. Alpha cells in the islets of Langerhans secrete gluaegon which releases sugar back into the blood. In this way the levels of serum sugars are regulated.

Most of this is under the direct control of the nervous system. When insulin is needed, it is the nerves which go to the pancreas, adrenals, and liver that control when the insulin is secreted and the proper amount to be absorbed by the tissues.

Suppose there is a disruption to the nerves which innervate these structures. If the nerve has been damaged, there is no way the body can coordinate the complicated series of events which occur. There are detectors in the alpha and beta cells in the pancreas which can determine how much excess sugar is present in the blood and then regulate how much insulin to release. The result can be diabetes mellitus. If the nerve has been damaged, there is no way the body can coordinate the complicated series of events which occur.

My friend, Dr. Daniel Murphy, had an interesting case. A lady, we'll call her Louise, had diabetes for 50 years (she was 55 at the time). Louise had been taking insulin by injection since she was five years old. She had never been to a chiropractor before. Dr. Murphy practices Chiropractic Biophysics, which means he tries to get the body into as perfect a posture as possible. He also sets the C1 vertebra so that it does not impinge on the brain stem.

Louise came to him for back pain, not diabetes. He adjusted her low back and then the area of her back which corresponds to the pancreas. He set her C1 vertebra precisely and sent her on her way. The next day she returned and told him that the strangest thing had happened. When she took her normal dose of insulin, she passed out; her husband had to revive her with a glucose shot. Somehow her pancreas had started producing its own insulin!

Louise called her son who happened to be a medical doctor and told him what had occurred. At the end of the conversation she said she didn't think she needed her insulin shots any more. He told her that was impossible and that she should simply start eating more sugar and keep taking the insulin shots! To this day, she eats a normal diet and no longer uses external doses of insulin.

Impossible you say? Consider this: when Louise was five years old she fell off a low brick wall, injuring her back. Ever since that incident she had problems with her blood sugar regulation.

This true story illustrates a valid point about chiropractic. If the dis–ease has been caused by a fall or some impact which has affected the position of the vertebrae, it is likely that resetting the vertebrae back to their original positions will correct the problem.

This case represents another important element: the son, who is an M.D., immediately wanted to control the symptoms. When the patient had too much sugar, it was reasonable to put her on insulin. Now that she had too much insulin, he wanted her to increase her sugar intake to compensate, rather than stop the medication she had been taking for so long.

It is tough to fight this kind of mind set. When drugs do not give the desired result, the situation and the patient should be re-evaluated, not just more drugs prescribed. Many of the M.D.'s I use in my referral network are those who prefer fewer drugs rather than more medication for their patients.

The body has an amazing capacity for regeneration, even in instances where the damage has gone on for long periods of time. However, it is possible that the organ, after years of altered nerve function, has atrophied and begun an early death. If this is the case, the organ or part of it, may have to be removed surgically if the patient has waited too long. This is the best reason of all to be checked by a chiropractor early and regularly.

If the diabetes is adult–onset and caused by a substantial weight gain, the patient may be managed not only by adjusting, but also through weight loss, exercise, diet and reduced stress. You see, we need other forms of therapy because these problems may be very complex. William A. Nelson, D.C., D.A.B.C.I., F.I.C.C. studied diabetes mellitus and its response to one type of chiropractic therapy.[50] His premise was that stress in these patients was a major factor in the symptomatology. He cites increased secretion of adrenal corticoid hormones in response to stress as what inhibited the activity of insulin.

He believed that chiropractic therapy would stabilize the nervous system's homeostasis via manipulation. The hypothesis was that a vasomotor imbalance caused by stress was causing circulatory problems seen in these two diabetics. After management in both cases, the conclusion was that the symptomatology was reduced with chiropractic care, although the diabetes was not "cured."

R. L. Dickinson, D.C. did a pilot study on the effects of chiropractic manipulation therapy on patients suffering from diabetes mellitus.[51] Thirty-one volunteer diabetics who had symptoms in the lower extremities, including numbness, coldness, discomfort and general weakness, coupled with discouragement for their future, were given chiropractic adjustments and interferential therapy. All patients reported some subjective improvement, between 50% and 100%. Several noted improvement in the days immediately following the adjustment. Although this was not a controlled study, its findings do lead to some important questions about how chiropractic can help control diabetes. The need for future research is evident.

4.   *Hypertension:* Hypertension is another word for high blood pressure (BP). This may include the systolic and/or the diastolic aspects of the BP. The systolic is the first number and is derived as the heart contracts and sends blood flowing through the arteries. The diastolic is the second number and is an indicator of the pressure in arteries when the heart is at rest. It is the diastolic which, when elevated, may be a more critical indicator of the condition.

Hypertension may be more of a symptom than an actual disease. In fact, the correct BP of 120/80 is only an average. Many of you have much lower and much higher BP which may never cause a problem. When your BP does elevate above its norm, it may be the correct response for that time and that condition. Controlling it with powerful and sometimes dangerous drugs may be to your detriment in the long run.[52]

Unlike many disorders of the body which can be traced back to the spine, there is no known spinal cause for the many types of hypertension. One controlled study was done with a small group of people whose blood pressure dropped significantly when their spines were adjusted chiropractically. The researchers used the activator adjusting instrument and found improvement in both the systolic (upper) and diastolic (lower) readings.

These subjects were compared to a control group and a placebo group, neither of which received any chiropractic adjustments or showed any improvement in blood pressure.[53] Other studies have shown the same results.[54] If the cause of the problem is the spine and nervous system, spinal adjusting may be the only solution, and no amount of medication will ever cure the problem. Instead it will only mask or control the symptoms.

In our office we have had many dramatic decreases in high blood pressure in patients with hypertension who happen to have back problems as well. In reality, we are not treating them for their hypertension, but rather the problems in their spine. However, just as in cases of asthma and other visceral disorders, these patients are showing remarkable improvements in their overall health with chiropractic care. At present we do not know the precise mechanisms by which these problems are being alleviated, but with further research we are learning how chiropractic can affect total health.

5.   *Cancer:* One of the most misunderstood areas of chiropractic is the ability of the chiropractor to affect the overall systemic health of the patient. You will recall that the first recorded chiropractic adjustment was not for back pain, but for deafness caused by one or more vertebrae being out of place and compressing the nerves leading to the hearing mechanism.

From then on, many people came to the early chiropractors for relief of different health problems and conditions. Many people found relief from migraines, diabetes, hypertension, gallbladder disease, colon troubles and, yes, even cancer.

The nerves control every function in the body. If vertebrae have been subluxated by even a small fall or accident, that target organ might not get the right amount of nutrients or nerve stimulation it needs in order to maintain proper function.

Let's say that the liver needs a certain quantity of blood running through it to stay healthy and properly flushed (the liver is a filter after all), and that this blood supply is regulated by the nervous system. The nervous system is protected by a batch of moveable bones in the back called vertebrae.

Let's suppose that one or more vertebrae slip or are knocked out of position and adversely affect the nerves leading to the blood vessels which control the flow to the liver. Now, part of the blood flow is cut off, and the liver which needs a constant supply of fresh blood to stay healthy (as do almost all parts of the body) is starved for oxygen. Tissue begins to die. This is a process called avascular necrosis. Avascular means without vascularity or blood, and necrosis means (tissue) death.

The toxins in the liver could also begin to back up because there is insufficient flushing due to decreased blood flow. Blood carries good things like nutrients and oxygen to the tissues and just as importantly, it carries bad things such as waste products and carbon dioxide away from the tissues. Each of these problems eventually could lead to a sick liver, cancer and/or death of the organ and the individual. A chiropractor will adjust the affected region in your back which corresponds to the liver, the blood vessels will open up, supply the organ with fresh blood in greater quantities, and now the PROBABILITY is higher that you will be healthy and disease-free.

There may be no chiropractic cure for cancer, only a hope of chiropractic prevention. Even this is not 100% guaranteed. If the individual smokes, has a terrible diet, gets little rest and is in constant turmoil, there is not much anyone (even a chiropractor) can do for that person unless there are other changes along the way. One reason that cancer has such a poor prognosis is that the patient will continue to do the very things that may have pre-disposed him to the disease in the first place.

Let's talk about the healing power of the body. When I was growing up, I knew some people who smoked every day, drank gallons of coffee, ate lots of greasy food and went to the bars every night (and some mornings too!). These people lived a long time in spite of all this abuse, not because of this lifestyle. My point is that all this abuse will eventually catch up to you. Why it doesn't kill you sooner is a testimonial to the recuperative powers of the body.

I have heard hundreds of stories from chiropractors, and testimonials from patients saying how chiropractic has cured their cancer, or at least put it into remission. The evidence is hard to refute. Patients who should be dead are still alive, and the only difference is that they started getting adjusted by a chiropractor. Most of the time it is the patient, not the chiropractor, who says they have been cured by chiropractic.

Unlike medical doctors, the chiropractor will not say the patient was being treated for cancer. We are adjusting subluxations in the back which have caused an interruption in nerve energy transmission to the organ(s) of that spinal region. Chiropractors are not medical doctors. We have much of the same training as far as diagnostic skills and physiology, but our philosophies and management regimes are radically different.

While the chiropractor tries to re-establish a normal physio-logic state in the patient and let the body heal itself, the M.D. tries to replace the body's normal functioning, at least temporarily, with chemicals which may have a healing effect. We both have our place in the health care system. Of course, if the cancer is in the advanced state, there may be nothing anyone can do. We would not try to give a patient false hope, nor would we try to take their hopes away.

It may never be too late to seek chiropractic care. Often we get our best success stories when all else has failed. That's usually when the patient is the most desperate, compliant and dedicated to care. The old saying is appropriate, "You never know until you try." I can tell you of several patients who probably would not be here today if they had not tried. Now that truly would have been a tragedy!

Imagine the mental anguish of being told you have cancer. Can you imagine what mental anguish is created just by the mere knowledge that you have a cancer? The stress of this news alone is enough to kill you! Even chemotherapy and radiation therapy, both of which are of questionable value, cause so much stress to the patient that their own validity has been called into question. Being sick as a dog and losing your hair does not seem to be a logical step towards health, regardless of what the drug companies tell you.

There is little evidence that you will live any longer by subjecting your body to these poisons. However, if you have lost a loved one to cancer and watched him or her go through the horrors of traditional therapy, do not reproach them or yourself for the decision.

Robert Mendelsohn, M.D. in *Confessions of a Medical Heretic*[55] says that modern cancer surgery is relatively useless. He cites Warren Cole at the University of Illinois who showed that when you examine the peripheral blood after the incision has been made, cancer cells have spread as a result of the surgery.

At present there is no cure for cancer, and neither the M.D.s nor the D.C.s can promise you one. You can increase the probability of extending your life if you embrace a complete change of lifestyle, including cleaning up your nervous system, diet, mental attitude, and resting the body so it can pull up all of its reserves to fight the cancer. It may be entirely necessary for the surgical removal of the tumor or even the entire organ if it has become so diseased that there is no hope of return to a healthy state.

I'm often asked if genetics play an important role in whether an individual gets cancer or not, and it's a good question. Emerging scientific evidence supports the theory that certain tissue and cell types passed on from one generation to the next may increase the likelihood that a person can get the disease. This is far different from the crack babies who inherit the addiction from their crack addict mothers through the placenta while in the womb. The latter is a direct passage of a toxin, not a change in genetics, as one may see with cancer carriers.

There is always the probability factor. If your parents had a certain type of cancer and you were their natural child, the probability would be higher that you would get the disease than your sister who was adopted at birth. What is lacking here is the importance of environmental factors.

If both of you ate the same high fat diet (i.e., fatty burgers, potato chips, fried foods, and lots of dairy products like creams and butter), smoked the same cigarettes, and yelled and screamed at each other the way your parents did, then your sister would have a high probability of developing cancer as well. Spinal or neurological weaknesses, such as scoliosis, are passed down also and could contribute to cancers by causing adverse changes in the nervous system.

Notice in the last paragraph I used the term "developing cancer." Many think or feel that cancer is something you catch, like a virus or bacterial infection. That would also indicate there was a magic bullet cure in the form of a pill, powder, or potion that you could take which would melt the cancer from your body. The idea behind the phrase "developing cancer" is that it takes a long time in most cases to get to the cancerous stage in tissue deformation.

A very good friend of mine was diagnosed with bladder cancer about sixteen years ago. Bladder cancer is often fatal within five years of its detection. He is still alive today and healthier than ever. At first, he would go in for a simple scraping procedure of the cancerous tissues of the inside of the bladder. As he was being treated he read the works of Linus Pauling, Ph.D. and others on the immune system and the important role vitamin C plays in overall health. My friend took massive doses of vitamins C, E, and A (he actually used beta carotene instead of A because it would not build up to a toxic level as quickly).

Tissue health is directly proportional to the amount of blood and oxygen which arrives at the cells. Vitamin E is a scavenger of what are known as free radicals which rob the cells of oxygen. By taking Vitamin E you get more oxygen to the tissues. Vitamin C is the builder of collagen which is the major component of the tissues (the concrete of the body, if you will). Vitamin A plays an important role in keeping the epithelial cells together and helps the body fight infection.

My friend currently lives a very healthy life, eats well, gets plenty of rest, and makes sure he laughs and plays his guitar every day. There is now no sign of cancer in his body.

You have only to read Norman Cousins' books for a good example of how laughter is therapeutic. Norman was diagnosed as having cancer. Of course, chemotherapy and radiation therapy were prescribed, neither of which has been proven to add to the quality or the length of life. The poisoning of the body may actually suppress the body's natural tendency toward health and healing.

Norman decided to take matters into his own hands. He also took vitamins, cleaned up his diet and life, and began to unleash the healing power of laughter. He bought movies such as the Marx Brothers old comedies and began to watch them every day. He laughed and laughed. He literally laughed his way back to good health!

This is an important lesson for us all. No matter how bad it gets, and it can be pretty bad at times, we should always find a way to break the cycle of depression. Laughter is one of nature's best cures.

Someone I like and respect very much is Mark Victor Hansen. He's an extraordinary motivational speaker, always up and happy. He has a great line he says to people who seem a little down. If he's passing you and asks how you are doing, most people will say "fine" or "great" when they are nothing of the sort. He smiles and says, "Well, if you are, you ought to tell your face about it!" I hope you were able to smile a little at that, a fitting end to a depressing subject like cancer.

6.   *AIDS:* As of this writing there is no cure for this terrible disease. Most of what is sold and prescribed is simply false hope. There has been little scientific evidence to support any mode of successful therapy. Some drugs may keep you alive longer, but none will eradicate the disease. As with many other diseases, we may never find a "cure."

It should be noted that many illnesses and diseases are known as "opportunistic infections." What this means is that the organism(s) hang around until there is an opportunity to invade the host — you. Usually this happens as the result of a compromised immune system.

AIDS, which stands for Acquired Immune Deficiency Syndrome, does not kill by itself. Instead, when a person has AIDS he or she is much more susceptible to organisms, such as bacteria and viruses, which are normally kept at bay by a healthy immune system. Many of us carry bacteria in our bodies, such as streptococcus in our throats, tuberculin in our lungs, and assorted bacteria in our urinary and digestive systems.

So why don't we all get strep throat, tuberculosis in our lungs, and yeast infections in our bladders? It is because we fight these diseases every moment of our lives through our immune system. It is automatic. You don't have to think about it or exercise it, and you don't have to control it. You only have to take care of it and watch over it.

If we don't get enough rest, eat nutritious foods in the right quantities, avoid mental anguish, get appropriate exercise and have a sound nervous system, we are likely to be attacked by otherwise neutralized bacteria. Now I must ask you again, where does health come from? It comes from within the body. Often the times in our lives when we have been the sickest are the times when we have been the most run down or stressed out.

Then along comes this terrible disease called AIDS. The reason it is so terrible is because it attacks the very thing which keeps us safe from every other disease known to man, our immune system. When AIDS has proliferated in the body, it allows other diseases to kill its host. The patient doesn't die from AIDS; he or she dies from the invasion of some other organism or disease.

You might ask what can chiropractic do for persons with HIV (Human Immunodefiency Virus) or AIDS conditions? Let me preface this by saying there is no hard scientific evidence that chiropractic can do anything for them. For that matter, there is no hard scientific evidence that any form of therapy can cure these diseases.

Let's analyze exactly what chiropractic does. It works on the immune system by helping to fortify and build up the body's resistance to diseases via the nervous system. It is no wonder many people affected with the AIDS virus are going to the chiropractor's office. Not because they are filled with the false hope of a miracle cure nor because they are clutching at straws, but because they believe in the sound principles being expressed by the chiropractor: your immune system is sick and chiropractic can help. It may not cure, but it can probably help.

The key ingredient is that the adjustment must be done specifically, properly, and at the correct levels of the spine by a doctor of chiropractic. A therapist, M.D. or your friend who can make some of your bones go "pop" by pushing or squeezing your back in a bear hug is not the answer. They may be "popping" the wrong ones and putting added pressure on the nerves that control your immune system. Nor can you do it yourself by "popping" your own neck and back. We know we can't cure AIDS, but we may be able to help—and we certainly can't hurt.

In the words of my good friend, Dr. Michael Schmidt, a chiropractor in San Francisco and the Academic Dean of Life Chiropractic College West, who teaches seminars on AIDS and the care of AIDS patients, "At this time we seem to be a profession who is making the HIV positive patient feel some relief, or at least like they are human and worth dignity. Our approach also makes a lot of sense to them. That's why I see so many people with AIDS in my practice. There are no side effects to the adjustment. Our adjustments optimize the body's potential for homeostasis and health."[56] All chiropractors want one thing—to stop this disease, whether it be in the form of a drug cure, the enhancement of the immune system, or a miracle of God.

7. *Psychogenic:* First, let me explain what psychogenic means. The pain is REAL. It is every bit as real as pain caused by an organic reason. However, psychogenic pain is caused by stresses the mind cannot or will not handle. It is unfortunate that Western science has denied those patients with psychogenic pains the empathy and concern they deserve. Nothing makes a patient angrier than hearing his or her trusted physician say, "It's all in your head." "Well, that may be true, doctor, but I didn't come to you for headaches, I came to you for low back pain!"

Any good practitioner, whether chiropractic or medical, will take the time to listen to your story. If there is a psychological component to the problem, a compassionate doctor should be able to handle it with dignity and proper protocol.

There is a saying that the organs cry the tears that the eyes refuse to shed. Stated simply, this means that those of us who were raised with the belief that you should internalize, or hold in your emotions, will suffer internal pain and emotional distress. This pain will often manifest itself in the soft tissues of the body, either the spine or the internal organs. Whether they show up first in the spine or the internal organs, be assured that they will migrate to and/or affect the other. As has been discussed in previous chapters, the two components are intimately connected.

One of my closest friends growing up was Michael. Michael was part of a very loving and close family before he was tragically killed at the age of 22 in a motor vehicle accident. Mike's mom, dad and grandparents were a second family to me while I was growing up. After Mike died, his family bravely got on with their lives.

Mike's mom probably suffered the most because she seemed to keep a lot of her pain inside. A few years after Mike was gone, she developed cancer that eventually took her life. To this day, I believe she lost her will to live because she lost Mike and kept much of the pain inside. It was especially hard for me because I saw the effect her death had on all of us who are still alive, especially her husband, other son, sister, and mother.

If I knew then what I know now, I would have tried very hard to get her into my office to be adjusted regularly (as her mom is) and try to get her into grief counseling, where she could have talked about her feelings toward Mike's passing.

If you know someone who has had a loss, as a loving friend or relative you will want to try to help them leave the past behind and stay with the world of the living—not just for their sake, but for the sake of those who are still here. Please refer them to a good chiropractor so their immune system has a fighting chance. One other good thing about chiropractors is that they usually have a very good ear for their patient's troubles. You may be saving a life.

In our office we always stress P.M.A., or Positive Mental Attitude. Many times patients come into my office who not only have physical problems but emotional problems as well. I have noticed that adjustments for people in this category don't hold as long nor as well as adjustments for other patients who are happier. I try not to let a patient leave my office without laughing or smiling at least once. It has been shown that laughter is incredibly therapeutic and healthy. In the section above on cancer this important concept was discussed. I have noticed that some patients leave the office after an adjustment feeling almost high; they are so happy and are feeling so good.

8. *Epilepsy:*   There are many forms of epilepsy. It is a disorder essentially characterized by recurring seizures, usually due to some type of neurological imbalance originating in the brain. The common classifications for these disorders are petit mal seizures

which are smaller and less severe and grand mal for larger and more severe seizures. Both types of seizures can result in loss of consciousness, severe bodily jerking, and often temporary loss of breathing.

Dr. Don Harrison in Alabama has had many patients with epilepsy. Once an eight-year-old girl, who was a patient of his and an epileptic, fell off the monkey bars at school and hit her head. She lapsed into a coma and was taken to a local hospital. After a few days the girl was still unconscious and deteriorating rapidly. The girl's parents asked Dr. Harrison to help.

He told them they needed to move her to his office so he could work on her, but the hospital would not release her. A few more days passed, and the parents were told there was little hope of recovery. They called Dr. Harrison who advised them merely to pick their daughter up and carry her out. "What will they do to us?" the mother asked. Dr. Harrison replied, "They will simply meet you at the door with all the proper forms to sign!" It happened just as he said.

When the parents brought the girl to Dr. Harrison he x-rayed her atlas, skull, and neck. She was still in a coma and could not hold her head up, so her father held her head in position until the film was taken. Dr. Harrison analyzed the x-ray, then placed the child on her side in the position he wanted. He put pressure on her atlas with the tip of the stylus of his upper cervical instrument. As the tip touched the atlas and put pressure in the correct direction, the girl's eyelids began to flutter. He delivered the thrust with the instrument and within five minutes the girl was fully conscious.

The girl is still doing fine to this day, although Dr. Harrison told me that one year after this happened the girl was playing on the monkey bars and fell off again, but this time she wasn't knocked unconscious. "Guess where they brought her first?" he asked me with a twinkle in his eye. "To you," I said. "Right," he responded "but I told them to take her to the hospital first to treat her broken arm and then bring her back for an adjustment!"

Robert J. Goodman, D.C. and John S. Mosby Jr., D.C., M.D., have reported in one patient that seizure disorder symptoms can be relieved by adjusting the occipito-atlanto-axial (C0-C1-C2) complex.[57] The patient was a five-year-old girl who, prior to being treated chiropractically, was experiencing 30 to 70 seizures per day. The Mayo Clinic determined the seizure types to be tonic, clonic, akinetic and grand mal. The diagnosis was Lennox-Gestaut Syndrome.

On July 18, 1989, the patient was taken for evaluation and care to the Palmer Chiropractic Clinic. The most notable finding of the chiropractic x-rays was that the patient's head, cervical, and upper thoracic spine would not line up over the patient's pelvis. The patient was adjusted only at the upper cervical region for three consecutive days. Very little change was noted the first day.

After the last adjustment made on the second day, the patient had no more seizures during the day. After the third day of adjusting, the patient had no more symptoms and postural changes were quite evident. In addition, a previously noted leg length discrepancy (one leg shorter than the other) was corrected; the legs became even after the adjustment. The report went on to say that fewer than 60 days after chiropractic care, the patient was reporting six or fewer seizures per day and on some days had no seizures. Her speech, which had diminished after the seizures started, began to return.

In this girl's case, the chiropractors were caring for the subluxations in her neck, not her symptoms of epilepsy. The case history was important in helping them with the diagnosis of the problem, yet they only managed the cervical misalignment. This proved effective in alleviating most of the symptoms. Once the cervicals were stabilized, no further improvement could be realized by continued adjusting. Other chiropractic studies have shown similar successes with chiropractic care.[58]

9. *Premenstrual Syndrome (PMS):* There are those who might argue that PMS is not a disease or even a dis–ease and should not be included in this section. I would suggest that these people have never experienced PMS on a first-hand basis. If they had they would have more empathy.

David E. Stude, D.C. quotes studies by R.V. Norris who called PMS "the syndrome that affects 5,000,000 American women," and also by G.E. Abraham who estimates that "at least $30 billion, 8% of the total wage cost, has been lost to U.S. industry because of PMS." He presented one case where a 35-year-old female, who suffered from PMS and had tried other forms of therapy, was helped by chiropractic adjustments.[59]

Many thousands of women are helped with their PMS symptoms by chiropractic adjustments. There have been many anecdotal reports and even some studies about the high success rate we experience. In our office there are several women who are on supportive care for their spine because most of their initial symptoms have been resolved. They often choose an appointment on the day of the month just before their PMS symptoms would normally occur. They had noticed a decrease of their symptoms when they were under corrective care and wondered if they would continue to be relatively symptom-free while on maintenance care.

Another study was done by Mark A. Wittler, D.C. who followed eleven women with PMS for four months. The women were between the ages of 23 and 42 and had not received chiropractic care in the previous six months. None were on medication during the study. In all cases they noticed improvements after chiropractic care.[60]

Both studies point out that they were not controlled trials, but they are important indicators that this problem is widespread, costly and could be helped with chiropractic care. They further suggest the need for future studies. It is up to you the patient to find out if your chiropractor has had experience helping patients suffering from PMS. If not, get a referral to a chiropractor who has such experience.

While I do not specialize in nutrition, I am a believer in the power of diet to affect your life.[61] Certain foods can produce or retard some of the ailments discussed in this chapter. For example, migraines can be triggered by chocolate, cheese and dairy products, fruits, alcohol, fatty foods, red meat and pork, tea, coffee, or seafood. A good diet to reduce stress is 60-70% vegetables, fruits, grains and cereals, 20–30% protein and 10–20% fat. A similar diet which avoids sugar can help manage rheumatoid arthritis. A diet which restricts meats can help with carpal tunnel syndrome. Reducing caffeine, salt, refined sugars and even dairy products can minimize PMS. In addition, vitamin and mineral supplements should be taken for specific health issues. Consult your chiropractor for concrete recommendations or referral to a nutrition specialist.

6

Different Techniques

Is there a method to this madness?

People will often tell me that they have been to different chiropractors over the years, and each doctor practiced differently. Even though the patient may have had the same complaint, each chiropractor had his or her own unique way of dealing with the problem. The good news was that their back and health usually improved regardless of the technique. Although potential patients may question this, it shows that there are many ways to solve a problem through chiropractic.

The "Standard of Care" established for the chiropractic profession has only recently been written (*The Mercy Guidelines*), and because it is relatively new its validity is still being tested. It is often difficult for the health consumer to know what type of chiropractor to choose.

Opening the Yellow Pages to the "chiropractic" heading in any major city will reveal many advertisements urging you to come here for neck relief or go there for a specialist in personal injury. This doctor does some mysterious thing called "The Palmer Method" or "Activator Only Practice," as though these things mean anything to the general health consumer. In fact, many chiropractors who do not advertise think some of these ads are downright embarrassing.

As mentioned previously, chiropractic is the art and science of adjusting the spine and joints of the body in such a way as to remove nerve interference and restore proper mobility and health. This is generally done by hand, but instruments such as the activator which deliver a quick, measured thrust work very well (some even claim they work better).

Every health profession has its "outsiders," someone who practices outside the realms of traditional methods. This is not meant to offend any doctor who practices these techniques or their patients who have benefitted from their therapies. Some people who have gone to chiropractic college (and some who haven't but claim they are doctors of chiropractic or their equivalent) have come up with some pretty bizarre forms of "treatment."

The problem is not the care provided, as long as there is no harm to the patient. The problem is that they call it "chiropractic." Waving crystals over a patient's head may provide, in your physician's opinion, maximum correction to the patient's spine, but it is not chiropractic. Crystals may cure cancer, a bad limp, or even hemorrhoids, but it is not chiropractic. Crystal use is neither taught in chiropractic colleges, nor is it researched or classified as a bona-fide technique. It may be therapeutic, but it is crystal therapy only, and nothing more.

My goal for this chapter is to describe briefly some of the main techniques of chiropractic and explain some of the specifics of each one. It is impossible to explain a particular technique fully; each would be a book in itself. It is not possible to list every technique performed in the chiropractic world. Many older techniques die out with their originators, and many new techniques are emerging every day to take their place.

However, if you are shopping around for a chiropractor and do not have a referral from a friend or family member, you may find this information useful. Additionally, if you are currently seeing a chiropractor and are not getting the results you hoped for, you may ask if he or she practices one of these other techniques. In Appendix D, I have also listed some people to contact who are leaders in each type of technique.

1. *Toggle Recoil:* Toggle recoil is one of the oldest forms of chiropractic adjustments, used and perfected by Drs. D.D. and B.J. Palmer and William Carver at the end of the nineteenth century and early part of this century. Emphasis is limited to the upper cervical (neck) only and consists of detailed analysis and adjusting of C1 and C2, the two top vertebrae. The idea behind any of the upper cervical techniques is that these vertebrae are the "master

vertebrae" of the body since they are the closest to the brain stem. Thus, all of the nerves of the body must pass through them first when exiting the brain. It is the upper cervical doctors of chiropractic who do most of the chiropractic miracles that are spoken of in this book.

The Toggle practitioner will often practice only the "Palmer Method" of chiropractic and will never adjust any vertebral segment below C2. These people are called "straight chiropractors" because of their strict adherence to Dr. B.J. Palmer's earliest teachings.

If you come in with a low back problem, they will adjust C1 or C2. If you come in with an elbow problem, they will do the same thing. This may sound ridiculous, but they get incredible

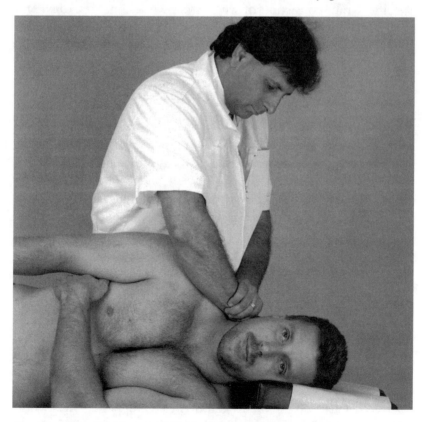

Toggle recoil is the oldest of the chiropractic techniques, utilized and perfected by D.D. Palmer, B.J. Palmer and William Carver.

results. In fact, when I get patients who are getting cold or flu symptoms, my usual protocol is to check the atlas to see if a toggle is called for. I have had several patients who have "miraculously" gotten over bad viruses by a toggle adjustment. Thousands of other chiropractors get these same results.

> My very first patient at the Life West Clinic was L, a nurse who is fond of working many shifts back to back. Once when she came in I could see she was overworked and about to get sick. I set her up on the table and toggled her C1 atlas. She immediately got very sleepy and, after her shift was over, went home and slept for over 14 hours. When she woke up, she felt great. This kind of finding deserves to be studied and researched.

The Toggle practitioner will probably take upper cervical specific x-rays consisting of what is known as a nasium view and possibly a vertex view. These are not standard medical views. They are specific to chiropractic and are designed to analyze the atlas in its three planes. Then the doctor will palpate the upper cervical region and, after studying the patient's x-rays, will determine the patient's "listing." This is approximately where and how the atlas has misaligned.

The adjustment is done with the patient lying on the side, head on a special headpiece that falls approximately $1/2$" when the right amount of pressure is placed on it. The chiropractor places the part of the heel of his or her hand that contains a tiny, pointed bone called the pisiform on the tip of the C1 or C2 vertebra. The thrust is quick and sudden with very little depth. It is just enough to cause the headpiece to fall. The correction is made by the doctor setting up the thrust vector in exactly the right direction and using just enough force to move the vertebra. When done correctly, it is one of the most powerful adjustments in chiropractic.

2.   *Biophysics:* Biophysics is a technique based on mathematical principles designed by Dr. Donald Harrison, M.S., D.C., Ph.D(c). As with Toggle, it is an upper cervical technique, but it also has the unique feature of bringing the patient's posture closer to that of a "perfectly balanced" spine. In addition to the upper cervical work, Dr. Harrison has designed and modified moves from other techniques to change the posture of the entire body.

The upper cervical adjusting, instead of being done on a toggle table, is done on a special table/instrument which delivers a precise amount of force in a precise direction to the atlas. In addition to this, there are levers and platforms which can raise or lower different parts of the body in order to compensate for postural defects.

For the rest of the body, Dr. Harrison has designed a table with a drop piece by the pelvis. The drop piece is designed for a specific reason. The part of the table that drops is under the vertebrae that are being adjusted. The doctor places his or her hands on the spine and presses down. The drop piece, spine, and doctor's hands fall suddenly at the same time. The table stops, the spine stops, but the hands keep going and the adjustment is made. There is no pain, and the adjustment is extremely precise.

Biophysics is also based on the work of Alf Breig, M.D., a Swedish neurosurgeon, who determined that as the spinal cord is stretched by improper posture the nerves are damaged, causing body dysfunction. In his book, *Adverse Mechanical Traction in the Central Nervous System*, he shows the results of stretching the head in different directions and the resulting damage to the nerves of the spine and beyond. It is this important work which shows the Biophysics practitioner exactly what is being accomplished as a patient's posture is being corrected.

An excellent example of this technique involves one of my favorite patients, H, who had a severe whiplash auto accident four years before seeing me. She had been treated by several medical doctors and chiropractors and had gotten some relief, but her overall condition had reached a plateau and wasn't getting any better.

H came in complaining of nausea and severe pressure over her right eye, coupled with headaches. X-rays and examination revealed many findings of posture abnormalities and soft tissue damage. One of the most important clinical findings for her case was the way her head deviated or translated forward and to the right, such that her chin rested over her right collar bone.

After a series of adjustments, her condition began to improve. The more her head began to center, the fewer symptoms she

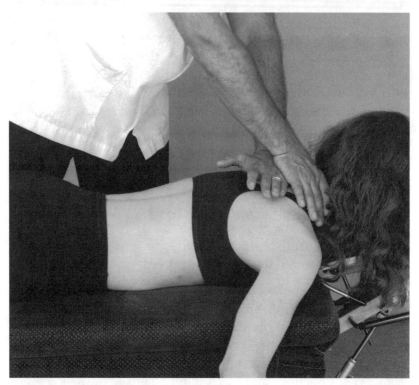

Biophysics adjusting of the cervical spine. This set up is for a person whose neck has flexed and translated forward.

experienced. She was also given a regimen of exercises which stretched her head into its proper position. This enabled her to control the symptoms at home between visits, rather than having to run back to our office in an acute state every day. She is now regaining some control over her life.

Biophysics is primarily the technique I practice to make the adjustment last longer and get a better overall correction, but I do some of the other techniques mentioned here for proper mobility of the spine and for controlling symptoms. The improvement in health is not only felt by the patient, but can also be measured and viewed by x-ray analysis during the course of care.

For lasting correction of your spine, I would urge you as a health consumer to make sure your chiropractor has attended at least one of the Biophysics seminars given by Dr. Don Harrison and Dr. Dan Murphy. I learned personally from the experts best qualified to teach it—the ones who designed the technique. There is really no other technique which changes a patient's posture to as noticeable a degree. This change may be necessary in order for your health to reach and stabilize at its optimum state.

3.   *NUCCA:*   NUCCA stands for National Upper Cervical Chiropractic Association. NUCCA people are what we call "squeezers." This is because they do everything the Toggle people do; however, instead of a quick adjustment which causes the headpiece of a table to drop, they simply touch the atlas with the lightest of force. Somehow they transfer the energy of their hands into the patient's C1 without moving their hands to any appreciable degree. And they get results! If before and after films are taken, you can actually see that the vertebrae have moved in spite of the fact that no audible (pop) is heard and no thrust is delivered.

One pioneer chiropractor who practiced and helped develop NUCCA was A.A. Wernsing, D.C. of Oakland, California. Dr. Wernsing practiced earlier in this century. In the 1930's and 1940's, he developed and refined the upper cervical specific x-rays that many chiropractors use. He also developed the actual NUCCA adjustment mentioned above (known to practitioners as the "triceps pull adjustment" because the doctor's triceps muscles are contracted when making a correct thrust). He was also instrumental in understanding the significance of measuring the degrees that the C1 atlas has become misaligned or subluxated.

One of the most famous NUCCA people is Dr. Albert Bertie, D.C. of Vancouver, British Columbia. Dr. Murphy likes to tell about his friend, another chiropractor, who took his young son to Dr. Bertie for ear infections. Since no one could help the chiropractor's son, surgery was being scheduled to insert tubes into the child's ears in order to help them drain, a common medical procedure. The chiropractor and his son went to see Dr. Bertie, who after careful analysis of the child, adjusted his atlas (C1) very precisely and sent him home. He also told the chiropractor not to let anyone else adjust the child's neck for at least a year. The ear infections cleared up immediately and never returned.

4.   *Diversified:*   Diversified is one of those techniques which borrows great ideas from many different practitioners and puts

them into a system it calls its own. This is not to imply theft, but rather a willingness to adapt to whatever works well and discard whatever does not. There is no philosophy or style which needs to be religiously adhered to, as in many other techniques.

Diversified is an osseous adjusting technique. This means a thrust is put into the vertebral joints of the spine, and there is actual movement of the subluxated vertebrae back into their correct positions. This is usually accompanied by an audible "pop" (technically called joint cavitation) as the joint releases carbon dioxide gas into the blood stream. There is usually a pleasant sensation and a sense of relief accompanied by a decrease of stiffness. There should be a great increase in joint range of motion following manipulation.

This technique is considered a "hard technique" because there is actual movement of the joint and joint cavitation. However, it is important to note that the thrust does not have to be

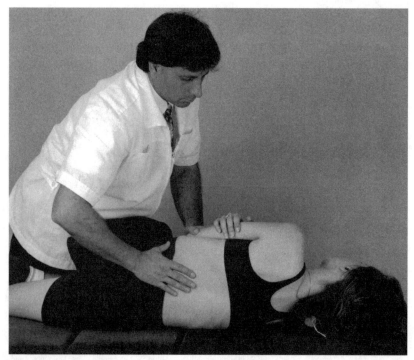

Diversified technique shown adjusting the lumbar spine.

done in a hard or painful manner. If done correctly, these techniques do not cause pain and are not dangerous.

As in Biophysics, Diversified is a full body adjusting technique which means every joint in the body can be adjusted when misaligned. However, unlike Biophysics, Diversified is not considered an upper cervical specific technique. Practitioners' analysis of the occiput-atlas-axis is based more on loss of range of motion, adhesions, and a specific misalignment rather than based on posture and measurement. Diversified is a very good technique for making locked joints move more freely and for relieving nerve pressure due to swelling.

5. *Biomechanics:* Biomechanics was started by Dr. Burl Pettybon of Oregon. Dr. Pettybon's work was a continuation of the work done by A.A. Wernsing, D.C. and others who were interested in upper cervical adjusting. Dr. Pettybon simply added the rest of the spine to the cervical region studied by these early pioneers and made up the Pettybon Spinal Model.[62]

This structural model showed that the spine exists in 30-60-90 degree angular triangles. Dr. Pettybon is responsible for modifying many Diversified adjustments into a form that is easier to use on larger and more difficult patients. Since Dr. Pettybon is still alive and practicing, it is to his credit that he is still changing and developing new and better ways to serve his patients.

6. *Thompson Drop Table:* Drs. Clay Thompson, Walter Pierce and Glen Stillwagon were instrumental in developing techniques and an important chiropractic tool known as the drop table (the table was discussed in the "Biophysics" section above). The drop table has been used to treat thousands of patients who, for one reason or another, cannot be adjusted in other ways such as with Diversified. It has also saved the backs of chiropractors who may be too small or unable to adjust some larger or stiffer patients. Patients who find themselves "tensing up" just prior to the thrust being delivered find it easier to be adjusted on the drop table.

The Drop Table technique uses many forms of analysis, one of which was developed by Dr. Derefield. Labels such as Derefield positive and Derefield negative are indicators of how the pelvis (either the hips or the sacrum) have misaligned. The analysis is based on doing repetitive leg length checks.

One leg, due to what is known as the bulboreticular inhibitory mechanism in the brain stem, will shorten or pull up more than the other leg, giving the appearance of a short leg on that side. This is due to muscle spasticity and is caused by vertebral subluxation. In the same way, the cervical spine is analyzed via leg checks.

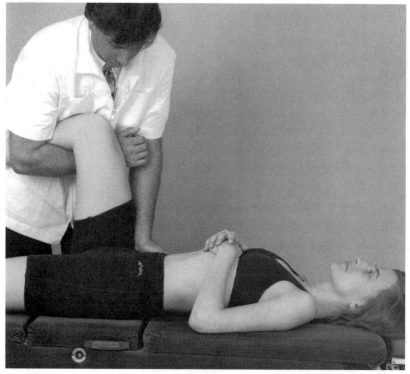

Drop table adjustment of the patient's right hip. These moves can be done very specifically and gently.

The drop pieces of the table are usually in the regions of the pelvis, the lumbars, the thoracics, and the cervicals. The patient is placed on the table when it is in the upright position and slowly lowered until it and the patient are horizontal. The analysis is done on the entire back using a variety of methods, and depending on the area to be adjusted, that part of the table is set. The thrust is delivered into the specific area of the spine and the set piece drops approximately $\frac{1}{2}$". There is no pain, and there may or may not be the sound of joint cavitation ("popping").

7.   *Activator:*   Activator Methods technique was co-developed by two chiropractors, Dr. Fuhr and Dr. Lee of Redwood Falls, MN. The Activator is a small hand-held instrument which delivers a measured thrust to the spine or whatever joint of the body is being adjusted. The great advantages Activator has over many techniques are its specificity, speed, and gentleness of delivery.

It is specific because the instrument head which delivers the thrust is small and may be placed right on the area and in the direction you wish to thrust. This makes it especially good for extremity work, where the bones in the hands and feet are tiny and difficult to move.

It delivers a thrust much faster than one can do manually, so it is impossible for the muscles of the patient to guard and resist. Finally, there is absolutely no pain. In fact, you may be wondering if the chiropractor has done anything at all. You will probably never hear the audible "pop" as with other techniques when the vertebrae move back into proper position. When done correctly, the Activator will move the vertebrae into the correct position and your symptoms should improve rapidly.

Another advantage Activator technique has is the analysis of the body. Dr. Fuhr and associates developed a system of checks and balances, coupled with scientifically reproducible results which are virtually indisputable. Dr. Fuhr himself has appeared before Congress in Washington, D.C., to address the issue of chiropractic health care in the United States. He is not only eloquent, but brings the science to back up his arguments. He is currently the director of the National Institute of Chiropractic Research (NICR). His organization has produced some of the most important chiropractic research to date.

The Activator is considered a soft or non-force technique, so its application can be for any patient at any age. The amount of the thrust can be regulated so specifically that the Activator is the method of choice for newborns, babies, infants, osteoporotic patients, the elderly or any patient who is in so much pain that manipulation is not an option.

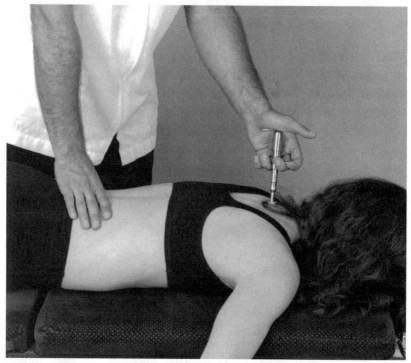

Activator adjustment of the upper thoracic vertebrae.

Many doctors have found they can use the Activator to adjust severely whiplashed patients who cannot turn their heads at all and are not candidates for osseous cervical manipulation. There is no torquing of the neck, which makes the Activator an excellent tool to use on patients who have some possible risk of stroke.

On the down side, some patients who have had a lot of trauma to their backs and a lot of fibrous adhesions may feel that the Activator does not move the joint enough to relieve their symptoms. They prefer a harder adjustment and usually seek out a doctor who does one of the more aggressive techniques. Of course, Dr. Fuhr would disagree and could show you data to prove his technique works as well as the harder adjustments. It is you, the patient, who must decide which technique works best for you.

8.   *Gonstead:* Clarence Gonstead, D.C. was one of the early pioneers of chiropractic and was an engineer who came up with many new and innovative techniques which helped thousands of people. He also taught his techniques to many doctors who, to this day, carry on his mission. Gonstead technique is taught in most of the major chiropractic colleges and remains one of the more popular ways to adjust the spine and extremities.

Gonstead technique is based on a detailed method of analyzing the spine using x-ray, palpation, skin temperature analyzers, and other methods to determine what is known as a "listing." A listing is the direction a vertebra has moved out of position with

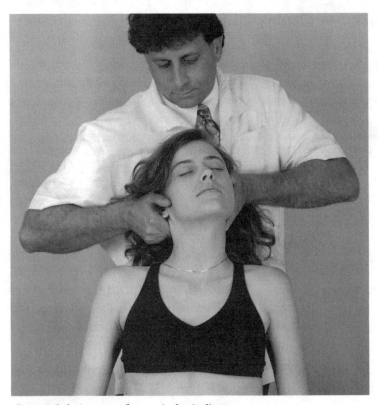

Gonstead chair set-up for cervical misalignment.

respect to the vertebra below. A typical listing for a vertebra in the middle of the back in the thoracic region might be PRS. This means that a particular vertebra has moved or subluxated posterior (backwards), right (the spinous process has rotated to the right), and superior (the transverse process on the right has moved up towards the head).

The Gonstead system of listing analysis and correction is one of the more popular chiropractic methods and is widely used.

9.   *Sacral Occipital Technique (SOT):* SOT is a very gentle technique developed by the late Dr. M.B. de Jarnette which explores the relationship between the sacrum (the triangular shaped bone at the base of the spine), the occiput (the skull), and the way the cerebrospinal fluid flows. The method looks at rotations and changes of the two structures and how misalignments of these areas affect the spine and the health of the body, especially the viscera (internal organs) of the body.

It relies on different classifications of blocking the hips and spine using special blocks as levers. This blocking is a slow, gentle way to stretch and retrain the ligaments of the body into their correct position. This work is somewhat similar to the work of Biophysics and other postural techniques, where a correction is made to the spine to change posture and permanently decrease or eliminate nerve interference.

10.   *Motion Palpation:* Motion Palpation is a technique for adjusting which incorporates what many chiropractors do every day as part of their analysis. Since most of us are concerned with making "stuck" joints move better, Motion Palpation directly lends itself to this. Essentially, the practitioner moves the particular spinal segment into the range of motion until it is restricted by subluxation. Then, by means of a quick thrust, he moves beyond this sticking point. It is a very good technique for restoring simple, normal range of motion to immobile joints. Motion palpaters are some of the smoothest adjusters in our profession.

11.   *B.E.S.T.:* B.E.S.T. stands for Bio-Energetic Synchronization Technique and was developed by Dr. M.T. Morter, Jr. of Arkansas. It is a non-forceful technique which tries

to remove nerve interference by lightly adjusting the spine and other areas of the body, including the abdomen, head, extremities, sternum, and sacrum.

Since this is a non-force technique, its proponents say it can be used safely on any patient including those who are in extreme pain, pregnant, elderly or newborns. Several of my colleagues say they get excellent, even unbelievable, results using B.E.S.T. with their patients. If your chiropractor wants to use this method for your condition, be sure to ask about the specifics of the technique.

12.   *Atlas Orthogonality:* Founder Roy W. Sweat, D.C., studied precise atlas (C1) listings in 1952, and originated Atlas Orthogonality in 1980. Like other cervical techniques, A.O. is based on precise measurements of the misalignment of the first cervical vertebrae. However, the instrument used is one of the most precise and uses the lightest force for subluxation correction in the profession.

Every year new techniques are developed in order to better serve our patients. When you ask your prospective chiropractor what techniques he or she uses, ask them to explain in detail what it is they do. Now that you have read this section, you may have some idea what is best suited for you. If you have further questions please refer to Appendix D. If you need more assistance please call or write me personally.

7

Who Needs Chiropractors? Everyone!

Chiropractic works by releasing the body's life-force energy. Unfortunately, we don't have a way to measure, either quantitatively or qualitatively, the concept of life-force.

— David Amaral, D.C.

Does everyone really need a chiropractor? Yes! Yes! Yes! If you have a spine, it's for you. If you've had a bad experience with a chiropractor (chiropractors are human after all), if you don't "believe in chiropractors" (we're not really ghosts), or even if you feel you are too sick or too far gone for care, it's for you. Doctors of chiropractic work on just about any living thing with a spine. Our specialty is people, of course!

When you have good consistent chiropractic health care, everybody wins. You win because you no longer have back pain, your joints and discs will not wear out as fast, and your overall systemic health and ability to fight disease improves. The chiropractor wins by earning a living doing something he or she loves and by getting daily rewards from patients who feel better and tell others about it.

Insurance companies and employers win because chiropractic care is usually cheaper and more effective for musculoskeletal related problems than medicine and surgery; people can go back to work faster and with less residual pain.[63] If employers save money, they can employ more people and this helps the economy. Finally, people who supply the chiropractors with everything from adjusting tables to typewriter paper, landlords, janitors, and carpenters will benefit from your business.

In addition to the different techniques discussed in the last chapter, many chiropractors practice certain specialties, just as doctors of medicine specialize. Some chiropractors specialize in children, athletes, the elderly, family care and pregnant women. There are those who see no patients but only read x-rays; these chiropractic radiologists have the same rigorous training and exam requirements as do medical radiologists. There are many chiropractors who only do examinations for insurance companies and evaluate patient management and care by other doctors.

There are chiropractors who teach and lecture for a living, and also those who write for national publications and health newsletters. Finally, there are chiropractors who work with veterinarians adjusting the spines of animals. Yes, animals have spines and nervous systems too! You can see that there is a wide variety of subdisciplines in the larger discipline of chiropractic. Now, let's look at some of the specialties in chiropractic.

1.   *Chiropractic and Children:* People who visit my office are often amazed at the number of children and babies we adjust. They usually ask, "What could a child possibly have wrong with their back?" Chiropractors adjust the spine for subluxations which cause more than just back pain.

Children have many diseases which are treated medically. Many of these diseases and sicknesses could be prevented if the child had a stronger immune system. In reality, it is the relative immaturity of a child's immune system which seems to cause the most problems. A misaligned vertebra or poor posture causing nerve interference in a child is magnified until the results cause more severe sickness in an adult. This often results in ear infections, high fevers and many visceral (organ) dysfunctions and diseases.

To look at what causes subluxations in a child we must examine the pregnancy of the mother and the delivery process. If a mother eats improperly, smokes, takes any kind of drugs including alcohol or caffeine, gets little rest or is highly stressed, she is compromising her baby's health.

The fetal heartbeat may actually increase each time the mother inhales a cigarette. The fetus is being starved for oxygen; the heart speeds up in response to compensate and send more blood to the organs. Remember that anything the mother takes into her body is passed through the placenta into the baby's body, including food, drugs, and cigarettes. The mother may not smoke at all, but can be exposed to second-hand smoke, which affects the baby.[64] All of these factors may have an adverse effect on the baby's developing nervous system and spine.

As the baby moves down the birth canal, he or she is compressed together. This is natural and usually okay, but many problems can result from the birth process. If the baby is too large or not in the proper position, or if the mother's pelvis is too small, there may be problems. As we study the way a woman's pelvis is put together, it is easy to see there may not be enough room for the baby to pass.

From a chiropractic perspective, as the mother's hips become misaligned or subluxated (one hip may move up and the other hip may move down), a torque is created in the pelvis which reduces its diameter. Instead of being at its maximum opening, it is narrower and may not allow full passage of the baby. There may be a fixation of one or both of the sacroiliac joints or pubic symphysis resulting in these joints not opening up. This may result in fetal stress and could cause several hours of hard labor.

The obstetrician may then elect to do a Caesarean section, a procedure where the mother's abdomen and uterus is opened surgically, and the baby is removed through the incision. In many cases this procedure, which may add days to the mother's stay in the hospital and months to her recovery, is often completely avoidable. It also greatly increases the risk to the mother, as would any major abdominal surgery.

Usually there is enough of the hormone relaxin (which causes the ligaments to expand) in the mother's body to allow for a normal delivery. However, if the pelvis or the spine is misaligned, there probably will be problems with the delivery. There will be more on this in the next section.

Another problem occurs when there is a subluxation in the lower spine, affecting the nerves which lead to the uterus and the other pelvic organs responsible for the birth process. As the pregnancy progresses and the mother carries increasing weight in the front, there is an increased load transferred to her back. When the back arches to compensate for the extra weight, increased pressure is placed on the discs, the facet joints and the nerves in the back (dorsal roots as they exit the intervertebral foramina). If this happens, there may not be normal communication between the brain and the rest of the organs, resulting in more problems with the delivery. Specifically, there are many hormones and neural impulses which are involved in the birth process. There is a relatively complicated set of events which goes on all through the pregnancy. These events speed up just before the actual contractions begin.

Many patients have their chiropractor in the delivery room with them as part of the health team to make sure all goes well (some even elect to have a home birth because the chiropractor is not allowed in the delivery room by the hospital).

If the baby has had trauma due to a difficult delivery, the doctor of chiropractic is there to adjust the newborn's back immediately. Yes, that's right, I said adjust your newborn's back! You may not realize it, but your baby has a tiny spine and nervous system which needs to be checked. I'm not talking about back pain, but rather your child's health.

During the delivery many obstetricians will put their hands on the newborn's head and with a strong pull and/or twist, yank the baby out. I don't intend to exaggerate, but in the course of an intense hard labor, even the doctor's adrenaline is bound to get elevated.

Even worse, if the mother is given drugs which hinder her ability to push and deliver the baby naturally, doctors may be forced to use forceps or suction on the baby's head. The newborn's neck is very delicate and any hard pulling is liable to cause tearing of the nerves in the neck and shoulders.

This is why we advocate the Bradley method of childbirth. It is based on natural birth processes without the use of drugs or medical intervention. It may be performed at home or in the hospital. I'm not suggesting the chiropractor do the delivery,

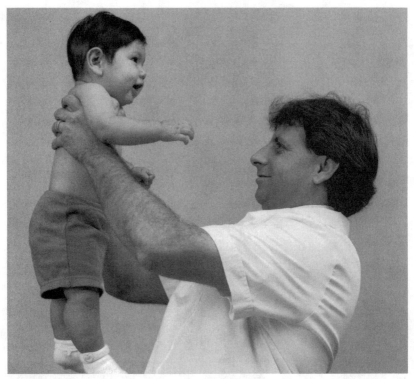

Checking the posture and spinal alignment of the baby.

even though in many states we are trained to do so. What I am suggesting is that after the pediatrician has checked all the baby's vital signs and all the baby's systems after delivery, the chiropractor should do an evaluation of the baby's spine and nervous system. If any adjustments need to be made to the spine, the chiropractor will be extremely gentle. It takes an imperceptible amount of force to move the newborn's spine into the proper position.

H. Biederman of Germany looked closely at how spinal adjusting helped babies suffering from birth trauma. He treated over 600 babies and found that infants who suffered from postural problems, sleeping disorders, extremity problems, facial swelling, painful necks, fevers of unknown origin, loss of range of motion of the hips and loss of appetite usually had a difficult birth.

The main problem he found was strained tissue at the base of the skull, termed suboccipital strain. In 50% of the cases manual adjusting was enough to control the symptoms, and in the other 50% some additional physiotherapy was also needed. He suggests that all babies suffering these symptoms, whether from a difficult birth or unknown causes, should seek adjustive therapy.[65]

An excellent review of the research was done in 1992 by Mark S. Gottlieb, a student at Logan College of Chiropractic. He looked at spinal cord, brain stem, and musculoskeletal injuries as a result of birth trauma. Some of the results of birth trauma include stillbirth, sudden infant death syndrome (SIDS), cerebral palsy, brachial plexus palsies, respiratory distress and ligament tears. In some cases these can lead to the death of the infant and, in other cases, there may be sleeping disorders, lowered immune functioning, colic, torticollis (neck muscle spasm) and visual and hearing disorders, among others.[66]

One of my instructors in chiropractic school, who is a chiropractor himself, told a story about the delivery of his twin boys. He was in charge of the delivery while the obstetrician and the nurse stood by in case anything went wrong. He had delivered the first boy and was waiting for the second baby. Suddenly the nurse said, "Doctor, your son has stopped breathing!" The chiropractor turned calmly, took his son out of her hands, ran his hands up to the baby's neck where it joins the skull, and lightly thrust his thumb into the first cervical vertebra. The newborn immediately flushed pink and started breathing deeply again. He handed the baby back to the startled nurse and the obstetrician and proceeded to deliver his other son.

Afterwards, the nurse and M.D. asked him what he had done. He really had a hard time remembering. He finally retraced his steps (he never once panicked) and figured out he had simply removed the pressure on his son's brain stem by adjusting the C1 vertebra. That vertebra is next to the area of the brain called the medulla oblongata which controls respiration.

Even when the chiropractor is not in the delivery room, it is a good idea to have the baby evaluated as soon as possible after leaving the hospital or birthing center. The chiropractor will not

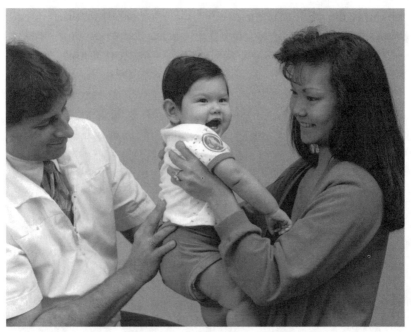

Adjusting a six-month old's spine can be gentle, specific and fun!

adjust your baby the same way he would adjust an adult; there is much less force needed.

What many chiropractors do is hold the infant up and check the level of the pelvis. If one side is higher than the other, we lay the baby down on his or her side and gently move the high hip down and the low hip up. We then have the parent hold the baby so that parent and baby are chest to chest. We run our fingers up the baby's spine feeling for vertebrae out of place and, if we find any, gently push them into place.

The last thing we do is check to see if the baby's C1 vertebra is in proper alignment. If not, we use our finger or a special instrument which delivers a tiny, measured thrust into the baby's C1. In reality, the thrust is barely perceptible; however, it does the job in a very quick and totally painless way.

This is the approach I use; however, many chiropractors may adjust babies differently. Personally, I like this method because it allows for the proper combination of subluxation removal and postural alignment that is needed for your baby's health. Indeed, many parents will bring their child to the chiropractor because they want the immune system to function at its highest level in order to fight off colds, flu, allergies, ear infections, and many of the diseases of childhood.

Many chiropractors say that children with ear infections make up a large part of their practice. If your child has an ear infection, he or she should be checked as soon as possible by a chiropractor who has had experience treating this problem. In our clinic we have seen several children who had sinus congestion and ear infections.

According to Jennifer Peet, D.C. ear infections are due to tension in the neck, causing a back–up in the normal fluid drainage of the lymphatics (including the inner ear).[67] If you were bacteria and you saw this fluid, you might think this would be a nice place to hang out for a while. The M.D. sees the bacteria as the problem and treats the symptom, which is the bacterial infection. He or she gives antibiotics which try to kill the bacteria. Unfortunately, all bacteria may not die and even if they do, different bacteria looking for a home might take their place. It is not uncommon for a child to be on several different antibiotics for months or even years as doctors try to find the magic drug to cure the symptom.

Alternatively, the chiropractor will look at the cause, tension in the neck producing a fluid back up. The adjustment will relax the neck and allow the lymphatics to drain naturally. Now there is no fluid for the bacteria to live in and the ear infection clears up almost immediately.

Why does this make so much sense? The parents of one child with ear infections who was adjusted in our clinic told us that their pediatrician was against chiropractic care, but the child's ear, nose and throat doctor (also an M.D.) was very much in favor of chiropractic care for infants.

Most children in our clinic respond in an average of two to three visits, even the ones already on antibiotics. However, if they have not had antibiotics and don't respond in a reasonably short time, they may need more invasive therapy. Antibiotics may be a necessary evil if it appears the infection may invade bone or blood, but this is usually the exception and not the rule. In most cases the child will respond to the chiropractic adjustment quicker and with fewer harmful side effects than with antibiotic therapy.

A 1989 study compared the health of 200 children under medical care with 200 under chiropractic care. The chiropractic children had fewer ear infections, fewer allergies, fewer cases of tonsillitis, and of course, less medical treatment such as antibiotic therapies, medications and vaccinations. The health of the children under chiropractic care was notably superior to that of children under medical care.[68]

For further information on antibiotic therapy and its limitations, I recommend you read the book *Beyond Antibiotics, Healthier Options for Families, 50 (or So) Ways to Boost Immunity and Avoid Antibiotics* by Drs. Michael A. Schmidt, Lendon H. Smith and Keith W. Sehnert, North Atlantic Books (1993).

Spinal care has been shown to help children with emotional, learning, behavioral and neurological problems. Pilot studies have confirmed clinical findings that chiropractic care has a positive effect on anxiety, inability to concentrate, low mental stamina, hyperactivity, discipline problems, and even low grades and low I.Q. After chiropractic care, grades improved, attention span increased, discipline problems diminished, energy and attitude improved, and neurological and other physical problems subsided. Chiropractic has the potential to become an important non-drug intervention for children with hyperactivity.[69]

As your child grows, it is important to keep a good record of treatments, visits to other doctors and any sicknesses. It may become apparent that your children will be healthier when they are adjusted regularly. Very often vertebrae are knocked out of place when children fall, are knocked over by the family dog, fall off the bike, play football or generally jar the spine. In short, anything which causes a blow directly to the spine, or through the rest of the body to the spine, can knock vertebrae out of alignment and affect the nerves at that level.

Further pressure is put on other regions of the spine which have now been placed at a biomechanical disadvantage by the primary vertebrae being out of place. The posture will be thrown out of proper alignment, the child may experience difficulty walking or running, or the muscles may begin to cramp after seemingly mild exertion.

If these symptoms are ignored, it is possible they may turn into serious health problems. As the immune system begins to diminish, the child may experience more flu, colds, and allergies. The body fights these with fevers, increased white blood cell production and general malaise which tries to force the child to slow down in order to heal.

The lymphatics, such as the tonsils, which are responsible for draining the dead white blood cells (pus), may begin to back up. As they repeatedly swell, an M.D. may want to remove them, but this does not solve the problem. The patient may need those tonsils someday. The problem is subluxation of the spine and the increasing immune deficiency the patient is suffering. The tonsils are simply doing their job.

Recall the osteopathic technique mentioned in the section on headaches. This is where you gently stroke with the fingers down the sides of the sternocleidomastoid muscle from the head down toward the heart. The lymphatic chains located there will drain when properly stimulated. This works especially well on children. Most medication merely controls symptoms.

As children grow, their spines may grow straight or crooked. When the back grows crookedly, it is called scoliosis. I have devoted a whole section to scoliosis in an earlier chapter. I hope you realize how important it is for you to look at your children's backs regularly, especially when they hit puberty where they experience several growth spurts. Look to see that hips and shoulders are level, spines are straight when upright and when they bend over at the waist, and finally that the head is on straight (no pun intended). From the side the head should sit up over the shoulders, and the shoulders should roll slightly forward, but not slouch. Finally, there should not be too much curve in the low back.

When your children are young, it is easy to watch how they grow up. However, when they get older, they may become more modest and you may have to resort to watching them at the beach or the pool. In any case, scoliosis screenings at the schools are not done often enough. I recommend they be done at least once every two months for the growing child. When unchecked, scoliosis will often get worse and may require chiropractic adjustments, braces, or even surgery in extreme cases.

If your child has behavioral problems including rages, belligerence, bed–wetting, hyperactivity, or is unable to sleep at night, it is possible, and quite probable, that he or she has a spinal and/or neurological problem. It's a shame that some family physicians will tell the parents to live with the problem, or make the parents

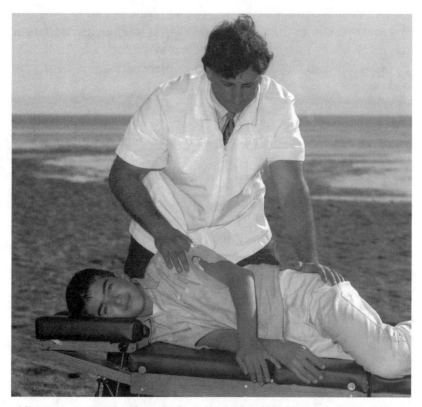

Adjusting a young "beachgoer" after a morning of hard beach activities. Most eleven year olds require very little care unless they have had some type of accident or have multiple health and/or back problems.

feel that they are not doing their job. The doctor may give drugs to suppress the symptoms but do nothing about the problem.

Even Dear Abby (Abigail Van Buren) has written on chiropractic solutions for bed-wetters. In her column in the *San Francisco Chronicle* on March 5, 1992, a mother wrote in telling about her two 15-year-old twins who were bed-wetters. Nothing helped until she took them to a chiropractor. Abby responded that she has had several hundred letters with the same message.

With behavior problems it is possible that the child has an imbalance between the sympathetic nervous system (the faster, fight-or-flight system) and the parasympathetic nervous system (responsible for digestion, sleep, and generally the slower more relaxed bodily functions).

In simple terms, it is the neurological balance between the two systems that allows the body to carry on daily activities. If there is too much sympathetic, the body will act at too high a level, similar to being on caffeine. If there is too much parasympathetic, the body is likely to be slow and lazy in its responses. The chiropractor can change with a few adjustments what no amount of scolding will ever accomplish. Your child will be able to do what is expected of him or her, and your relationship will not suffer.

As a teenager, your child will go through many changes, both emotionally and physically. They need straight spines and healthy organs, if for nothing else than to process the vast quantities of junk food they force into their bodies. On the chance you have been able to instill in them a love for proper nutrition and they are fortunate enough to have a healthy spine, they'll form habits which will keep them pain-free and healthy all their lives. The moral here is that child chiropractic patients are always "well-adjusted."

2. ***Chiropractic and Pregnancy:*** By now you should have some concept of how important good chiropractic care is to your overall health. Your back pain will disappear or diminish and more importantly, your overall health will take a quantum leap forward. Pregnant patients present special challenges to the clinician. Robert S. Mendelsohn, M.D. in *Confessions of a Medical Heretic*

points out the dangers of many drugs and states that every drug should be approached with suspicion.

He cautions that pregnant women and their babies are better off to avoid all drugs completely. He says that even though a drug may not have any side effects on you, it may be doing a great deal of harm to your developing fetus. It is not unusual to find out the damaging side effects of drugs only after they have been on the market for a long time. However, if you or your baby's life is at stake, you may have to chance the side effects rather than risk your lives.

In spite of the evidence (mostly clinical, but also some controlled studies), it is interesting that many obstetricians overlook chiropractic care for their mothers-to-be. When we think about the radical changes the body goes through during pregnancy, it only makes sense to have a good chiropractor as part of the health care team.

Physically, the mother is getting bigger and bigger. Her low back is forced to carry increasing weight at a lower and lower angle. This causes the low back to arch more than it is accustomed to. If you think back to our early model, the lumbars should be at around a 40 degree angle. It has been established that women in their third trimester of pregnancy can have as much as a 90 degree angle.

The longer and bigger the lever, the more force at the fulcrum, in this case the back. The facets jam up causing local, deep pain. The nerve holes (intervertebral foramina or IVFs) shrink, causing swelling which exerts pressure on the nerves. This can cause pain down the legs, also known as sciatica. The discs between the vertebrae in the low back are compressed more than usual in the back, causing increased wear and tear. The increased pain to the mother can cause increased stress, which is not good for the baby's health. Finally, the fact that the nerves are being compressed means that their target organs are not getting the proper signals from the brain, which could cause a decrease in blood flow to or from that organ, including the uterus, which is supporting your future child.[70]

There needs to be an uninterrupted channel of communication as the brain and body begin the birth process. The spinal cord is the communication channel. If there is abnormal stress on the nerves, especially the nerves in the low back which go to the uterus through the autonomic nervous system, almost anything can go wrong.

I'm not recommending that you abandon your midwife or obstetrician or anyone else, but I am suggesting that you see a chiropractor during your pregnancy and immediately before you deliver. He or she can adjust your back and pelvis to make sure you have the best possible spinal alignment in order to ensure not only your health and the health of your baby, but possibly an easier delivery. In our office, our pregnant patients average approximately six-hour deliveries. This is typical throughout the profession. The national average for first time mothers is 12-14 hours and second time mothers is 8-10 hours. 20 or more hour labors are not uncommon without chiropractic care.

Another problem encountered during pregnancy is the increase in size of the mother's breasts with the beginning of the cycle of milk production. Increased pressure is put on the middle of the back; the dynamics of balance change throughout the spine. If the spine was previously healthy and straight, then there will probably be few problems. If the mom has a bad back to begin with, the pregnancy will only make matters worse.

We have also noticed increased problems with the mother's neck and upper back as she nurses her baby. She is generally looking down while nursing and putting increased strain on her neck and upper back musculature. Holding one position for longer than 20 minutes will generally stretch and strain her ligaments. We recommend she use pillows to help support her child and every few minutes look up and stretch her neck. This will greatly help the soft tissue structures.

One final concept with pregnancy is the hormonal changes that take place. The hormone relaxin is released, which effectively softens up all the ligaments in the body in anticipation of their impending stretch. This causes the vertebrae to lose their normal position much more readily and allows problems to occur more frequently.

Taking this one step further, post partum is one of the best times to be under chiropractic care. As the relaxin subsides, the tissues harden. When you are adjusted, the chiropractor is effectively molding your back into its correct shape, one which will serve you better and remain much stronger.

3.   *Chiropractic and Athletes:* The story goes that after Greg Louganis hit the back of his head on the platform during the 1988 Olympic diving competition he went to his team chiropractor and received an adjustment of his cervical spine. He then went on to win the gold medal in that event. Greg Louganis knew that with all his body weight falling on his neck that something had to be knocked out of place, probably several vertebrae. His chiropractor at the Olympics was Dr. Jan Corwin of Oakland, California, who is an expert on athletic injuries. Although there were many medical doctors at the Olympics, most were not very busy, unless there was a major trauma to an athlete. However, Dr. Corwin found himself constantly busy as he adjusted one athlete after another for everything from back pain to foot problems.[71]

Just prior to the 1990 Super Bowl game, Joe Montana, quarterback for the world champion San Francisco 49ers, was adjusted on national TV by his personal chiropractor, Nick Athens, who had flown to New Orleans to take care of several of the team members. When Dr. Athens arrived at the hotel where the players were staying, he was immediately handed a huge stack of messages from several players to see each one of them for an adjustment.

Roger Craig, the award-winning running back who played for the 49ers, has stated that the Monday after a hard hitting football game, he ices his body to keep the swelling down and gets a deep tissue massage. On Tuesday, he goes to Dr. Athens and gets his adjustment. On Wednesday, he is running at full speed in practice. He knows that several vertebrae are knocked out of place during each football game.

What do the 49ers and Greg Louganis know that many athletes don't know? The secret to winning or doing your best at any sport is making sure your body is performing at top physical condition. The nerves to the muscles not only cause the muscle to contract and deliver motion, but are also responsible for controlling the amount of blood into that muscle and the rate the muscle repairs itself following stress. The only way a nerve can work properly is by having an open and unencumbered passageway to and from the brain.

If a vertebra or group of vertebrae have been traumatized and restricted in motion and/or pressure has been placed on that corresponding nerve, it is impossible for the muscle to receive the proper amount of blood, nutrients, or stimulation it needs to repair and nourish itself.

Very often when in the gym or out running, I see "serious" athletes working very hard on their bodies to get the look and the feel that they want. The sad thing is they are often not achieving their peak condition. It's not that they are not putting in the effort, far from it. Their body is not recovering and they, in their desire to improve rapidly, work out on already damaged tissue causing further stress and strain.

This is almost a catch–22 situation. What the muscle needs is rest, nourishment and especially a sound nerve supply. I often ask them who their family chiropractor is, and they seldom have one. I tell them that most of the top athletes have a chiropractor, and I try to point out that if they expect maximum performance out of their bodies they have to give themselves a maximum chance of recovery and a clear nervous system.

An excellent study was done by Anthony Lauro, D.C. and Brian Mouch, D.C. comparing the athletic performance of athletes under chiropractic care versus those not receiving adjustments.[72] They took 50 asymptomatic athletes and adjusted half of them and did not adjust the other 25 (the control group). They looked at tests of agility, perception, power, speed of reaction and speed of movement. These tests measured characteristics which were more inborn and minimally affected by strength or cardiovascular work.

After six weeks of adjusting, the athletes were all retested. In the control group of non-adjusted athletes eight out of eleven improved their performance, but by less than 3%, or an Index of Average Athletic Improvement (IAAI) of 4.5%. This improvement was attributed to a second opportunity to do the same test. In the test group of chiropractically adjusted athletes all improved their performance by greater than 3%, or an IAAI of 10.5%.

The experimenters went one step further. They had released the control group but decided to retest the chiropractic group after another six weeks. They found that the group's performance level had increased again to a IAAI level of 16.7%! According to Malik Slosberg, M.S., D.C., of Life Chiropractic College West, this study shows chiropractic care goes way beyond pain relief. Chiropractic care can actually improve athletic ability, even for athletes who have no obvious back problems at all.

Golf: Golfers are a classic example of a group of athletes who often have bad backs. I taught golf many years ago and have a good understanding of the nature of the golf swing. One good book I used to teach from was *Ben Hogan's Five Lessons: The Modern Fundamentals of Golf* with Herbert Warren Wind and artist Anthony Ravielli.[73] This book contains an excellent set of drawings of the proper backswing, downswing and follow through.

The maximum amount of tension to the back is present at the top of the backswing and the beginning of the downswing, which is necessary to create enough club head speed to drive the ball down the fairway. The drawings show the golfer completely torqued, with his knees starting to drive forward toward the target, but with his back and shoulders still completely turned backwards! This illustrates the tremendous "wind up" a golfer must do throughout the many swings he or she takes (these days some of us take more swings than we used to!).

I adjust many golfers for low back pain, in addition to neck, mid-back, elbow and shoulder pain. These patients seem to lose fewer days on the golf course due to bad backs than they did before becoming chiropractic patients. The real tribute to this is the many touring golf pros who have their own personal chiropractor and referral lists of other chiropractors in the many different states they visit while on tour.

Body Building: People who lift weights on a regular basis were often scorned and even laughed at in the past, but I don't know many people who laugh at Arnold Schwarzenegger. He has done for weight lifting what Arnold Palmer did for golf—brought it to the masses and made it into a popular sport for everyone. For a healthy back, some proper weightlifting on a regular basis is crucial. It used to be thought that people who lifted weights were stiff and rigid due to their strong muscles. Today we know that a strong muscle does contract stronger, but it also relaxes better!

There has recently been a great increase in the number of bodybuilders and powerlifters seeking chiropractic care. Most have found they are making greater gains in strength, size and recovery when they are adjusted regularly. Some are also winning more contests.

Even athletes who lift weights for enhancement of their own sport realize the need for good gains and recovery times. Most sports put tremendous physical strain on the athlete's body. These individuals usually want all the help they can get in attaining their goals.

Two famous bodybuilders are also chiropractors, Dr. Franco Columbu (winner of Mr. Italy, Mr. Europe, Mr. International, Mr. World, and two time winner of the Mr. Olympia title) and Dr. Tom Deters, Editor-in-Chief and Associate Publisher of *Joe Weider's Muscle and Fitness Magazine*, the world's number one fitness magazine. Dr. Columbu maintains a private practice in the Los Angeles area, while Dr. Deters, who holds licenses in three states, is an extensive publisher, author, educator, and television commentator for many professional bodybuilding events.

Dr. Columbu has also authored several publications on chiropractic, sports, and bodybuilding and has appeared on television and in many motion pictures, including "Pumping Iron," "Terminator," "Stay Hungry," "Conan–The Barbarian," and others. Both of these gentlemen were honored in 1993 at the Arnold

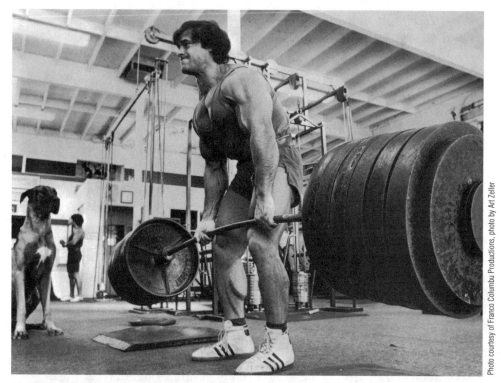

Dr. Franco Columbu dead lifting 750 lbs!!

(Schwarzenegger) Classic by the International Chiropractic Association for contributions to their profession.

Every month *Muscle and Fitness* magazine has excellent articles on fitness and health, and several times per year they publish a column entitled "Back Corner," (previously "Backtalk") which is devoted to helping their readers maintain a strong and healthy back. The March, 1992 issue carried an excellent series of articles by Dr. Deters and others about back pain and how exercise and therapy, including chiropractic, can help. He also explained how the back may become damaged during bodybuilding and how this can be avoided.

In the magazine's section on injuries, Dr. Deters and Jeff Everson, L.P.T. tell how bodybuilders often injure themselves. They state, "Bodybuilding is generally a very safe sport with few injuries. Better yet, injuries that do occur are usually preventable.

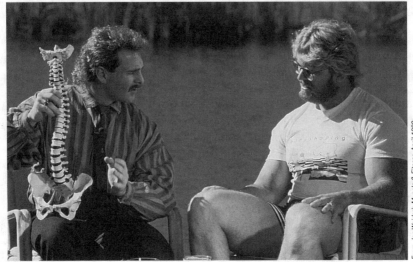

From *Joe Weider's Muscle & Fitness*, April 1992;
Photo by Robert Reiff Courtesy of Weider Publications, Inc.

Tom Deters, D.C. (L) explains the benefits of chiropractic and bodybuilding to Jeff Everson (R) for ESPN, the cable TV sports channel.

The most common cause of lower back injury in bodybuilding is improper lifting technique. An unstable starting position and bouncing or jerking the weight at any point throughout the movement practically guarantee an injury.

"These bastardizations of the Weider Cheating Principle can create rapid and extreme stress on muscles, ligaments and discs. Bouncing or jerking during the lift allows momentum to create even greater loads since momentum can magnify a weight many times. If you were to drop a two-pound weight off a tall building, the weight would still weigh two pounds, but since it was moving so fast its force would be much greater. The same thing applies if you do a bench press and bounce it off your chest. A 200-pound barbell can then easily transmit 400 pounds of stress to the shoulder joint.

"Keep in mind that a sudden movement in the wrong direction is likelier to cause an injury than a heavy deadlift done with good form. Most lower back injuries occur when you are in a flexed or hyperextended position and then twist. This means that you need to pay close attention to your technique when you put those dumbbells back on the rack. For the same reason we want to avoid over-rotating our lower backs with twisting movements; you see many people doing this with a broom handle across their shoulders. The lower back is designed to rotate only 30 degrees. Any more than that and you stress the discs and ligaments."[74]

My good friend and colleague Dr. Ronald Fritz of San Diego, California, has lifted weights for years and takes care of many bodybuilders and powerlifters. He stresses to them the importance of proper body mechanics, rest, nutrition and, most important of all, getting their spines adjusted and remaining free of subluxations. They have found that on average, they can lift heavier weights with increased flexibility and reduced recuperation time

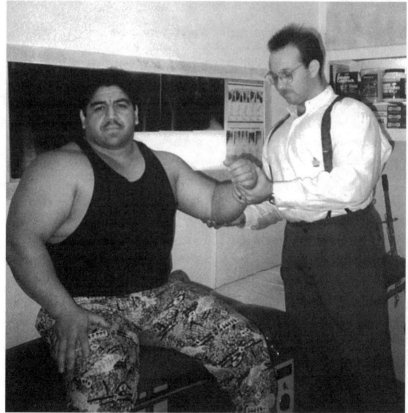

Photo courtesy of Dr. Ronald Fritz

Ronald Fritz, D.C., C.C.S.P. checking Alex Estrada's arm. Alex credits regular chiropractic care as contributing to his success.

when they are adjusted regularly — usually once or twice per week.[75]

Dr. Fritz takes care of Alex Estrada who is currently ranked as one of the top lifters with the American Drug-Free Powerlifting Federation. Alex and many other elite powerlifters use chiropractic care routinely to enhance performance.

4. *Chiropractic, Police and Firefighters:* Law enforcement, fire fighting and rescue work are some of the toughest, most physically demanding jobs in the world. In addition to having to keep themselves in reasonably good physical shape, these professionals have to be mentally alert at all times. Their actions could save or cost a life in many situations, and they are under constant physical and mental stress. They cannot stop for back pain or other physical ailments.

Many of them have their own chiropractors who keep them going. They know they can perform their jobs better when they are relaxed and pain-free; chiropractic care helps keep them this way. My friend and colleague, Dr. Ethan Feldman of Berkeley, California presents lectures to law enforcement agencies concerning on-the-job care of the back. He tries to focus on prevention of back problems. He told me he is still trying to identify a way to teach how to tackle a suspect in an "ergonomically correct" manner!

These jobs are further complicated when you realize these professionals cannot take any drugs while on duty. Even over-the-counter drugs such as painkillers or antihistamines could slow down their reflexes enough to endanger their partner's life, their own, or even the public's. For them, chiropractic is the logical choice.

5. *Chiropractic and Nurses:* Even though this section is devoted to one of my favorite groups of patients, medical nurses, many of the principles here apply to other professionals who are under a great deal of job-related stress, hold their arms up for extended periods of time and must lift weights at bad angles.

One of the reasons nurses are my favorite patients is that my mother is a nurse. She has set an example for me by always being at the service of other people, and this is what has brought her true happiness. I have observed this joy in service to others in many doctors and nurses who love to serve their patients. Some of the happiest nurses, chiropractors and other physicians I know are the ones who serve a great number of patients.

The chiropractors I know who have risen to the top of our profession are those people who have had very large practices and have gotten great rewards for their services, but they are also the ones who have "washed the most feet" as the saying goes. I cannot think of one professional nurse who is not worth his or her weight in gold for the service they provide their patients. They deserve to have their spines and health cared for and preserved.

There are three reasons why nurses make great patients:

1.   They are bright, intelligent, and understand the body. Chiropractors do not have to work very hard to explain to them what they already know about anatomy and physiology.

2.   They are in contact with a large patient population and are eager to see more patients get well. Once they understand the nature of chiropractic they want to get these suffering patients in to get their spines checked. Then they want to bring in their families and friends.

3.   Due to the nature of their job, in which there are great physical demands, they are always throwing their backs out and will be patients for life. They understand drug therapy has its place in pain control, but if they have misaligned vertebrae and nerve dysfunction, they want to be adjusted. They know mechanical problems require mechanical solutions and chemical problems require chemical solutions. If they are poisoned, they will get a chemical solution — drugs, but if their back hurts, the mechanical solution is to be adjusted by a chiropractor.

When you watch nurses work, as I have done for a number of years, you can begin to appreciate the enormous amount of physical, mental and emotional stress they are constantly under. They have to move large patients around all day, make quick, life-saving decisions and deal with concerned families and patient deaths on a routine basis.

It is not uncommon for nurses to get very attached to their patients, only to lose them in the end, despite their heroic efforts. Often, they must take orders from seemingly gruff doctors who are also under a great deal of stress and may not always be giving the right orders for a patient. The nurses must either do what they have been told or confront the doctor with a better suggestion. This creates a very stressful environment.

Many of the nurses I care for tell me that my office is the "eye of the storm" as they leave their patients and go home to care for their family, or vice versa. If there was ever a profession under-paid and overworked it is the nursing field.

6.   ***Chiropractic and Construction Workers:*** Just as with the other groups previously discussed, heavy equipment operators and construction workers are in danger of on-the-job back injury con-stantly. One of my patients who drives a bulldozer over rocky, rough terrain says he can feel his back go out whenever he hits a big rock. After a short time the pain really sets in. As long as he continues to do this job, he needs chiropractic care.

Often it is like a tackle football game, where the spine is the subject of constant impact from a variety of sources and directions. Some may just ignore the problem until it sidelines them for days, weeks or even months. Others try to get it taken care of as soon as possible in order not to miss a day's work and pay.

Even sanitation engineers subject their backs to constant strain and stress by lifting, pulling and pushing. Some use dollies to roll the garbage cans around, but others still carry the garbage cans on their back. Both groups, however, still have to do all the lifting to empty the trash into the back of the truck. They also swear by their chiropractors and say the cost of care is definitely worth being able to work relatively pain-free.

7.   ***Chiropractic and Wise, Honored, Experienced People —
(The Elderly):*** If you are fortunate enough, you get to become a member of this group of people. The subject of geriatrics is an ever expanding one as the population of the world gets older. People

today live longer than at any point in our recorded history, but are they living healthier, more dignified lives? This is debatable.

In the United States we keep a growing watch on one particular group of people that we have closely studied — the Baby Boomers. This is the group (of which I am a part) born between 1945 and 1963, also known as the post–war generation. Although far from elderly, this population is growing older. There is growing concern among all of us for a better way to stay healthy. I'm not implying we baby boomers are ready for the rocking chair yet, but all of us are getting older.

Whether we like it or not, we must admit we are growing older. Our backs, organs and immune systems are aging. This puts us at risk for many health problems we thought belonged only to our parents. Further, since our generation has become leaders and trendsetters we demand better choices, and for us chiropractic care is the new realm of health care. We know drugs only mask the symptoms and allow the underlying problems to get worse with time.

Another group with special "challenges" is the generation(s) before the Baby Boomers — the true senior citizens. These people should and do have a special place in our hearts, for it is they who fed us and clothed us and kept us safe for all those years. Now it is their payback time, and many are being drastically shortchanged.

As people age many things happen to their bodies. Their old and trusted friend begins to turn on them and stops working as well as it once did. The bones begin to weaken as they lose calcium. This is known as osteoporosis. The blood vessels begin to wither and either get weaker or plug up with fatty plaque (atherosclerosis, a stage of arteriosclerosis). This has the effect of increasing blood pressure (hypertension). Increased blood pressure can cause many health problems, such as dizziness, blindness and headaches.

The shock absorber disc pads in the spine begin to degenerate and can, without chiropractic care, break apart and cause the bodies of the vertebrae to fuse. This in turn, causes subluxations which can change the function of the nerves which exit the spine on each side and at each level. To reiterate an earlier point, when there are vertebral subluxations and/or dysfunction of the nerves, the blood vessels which go to the organs at the ends of those nerves begin to constrict (get smaller). There is less blood delivered to the organs at the affected level causing an early death of the tissues of that particular organ.

When the vertebrae are adjusted back into the proper position, there is an immediate increase in the size of the blood vessel and more blood is delivered to the organ. This is good!! This is really what chiropractic is all about.

Other problems the elderly face include decreases in energy, greater depression and pains in the joints such as arthritis. Chiropractic can help with all of these conditions. Life is about motion in the body and in the mind. Life also depends on good blood flow.

A chiropractor's job is to keep everything moving in the body as it is designed to move. If a joint is moving too much and wearing down too rapidly, we need to reduce its motion. If something is stuck in place, we need to free it up, and reestablish normal motion. Motion is life and life is motion! Overcoming poor posture helps hold the adjusted vertebrae in their proper positions.

Bill Ruch, D.C. of Oakland, California has some senior citizen patients who need extensive posture work. He has noticed that they have a tendency to droop forward at the shoulders and bend forward in the center of the back. In order to counteract this, he sits behind them. As they inhale deeply he puts pressure on their backs with his hands. He then crosses their arms in front of them and lifts their arms up as their chest expands. This allows their back to straighten temporarily and the ligaments to stretch. Often the patients will tell Dr. Ruch that they feel they are standing straighter; the sink or the counter at home looks further away as they stand upright.

In addition to this, Dr. Ruch's patients, as well as my own, report they are able to breathe deeper and a little easier as they become straighter. In part, this is due to the increased volume inside their chest.

I have one patient who is a professional singer with two albums to his credit. He comes in for care whenever his lungs constrict and he can't hit certain notes as he sings. These findings indicate that if there is a greater exchange of air going on, this type of therapy might merit some studies on the long-term benefits to the overall health of the patient.

8.   *Chiropractic and the Military:* Recently there has been a push to get chiropractors into the military as commissioned officers. The logic behind this is that our education is on a par with medicine (we are doctors like our medical counterparts), and we are the best equipped to handle soft tissue injuries to the spine as a result of military activities.

Chiropractors are the first to admit that our services may not be as important in times of war as that of a surgeon, but if a soldier cannot function due to back problems we are needed. Even in times of peace we may be most urgently needed because there is a greater likelihood of disability due to non-combat back injuries. Ask anyone who has been in sick bay due to a back condition, and they will tell you it can be as tough as being shot!

People who have been under chiropractic care prior to going into the military are especially at a disadvantage after they join. Once they are in the military, they can no longer get the chiropractic care they want and need because it is not part of the military. Some say their headaches and back pain return without regular chiropractic maintenance care. This is unfortunate because it can diminish their potential as a soldier.

Let's focus on one job in the military where the back may feel stresses and strains—the duties of a fighter pilot. In the cockpit of any supersonic jet a pilot's body may be subject to several times the force of gravity (called "G" Forces). In the movie "TOP GUN," a bemused Tom Cruise describes to an incredulous Kelly McGillis how he did a 4G negative push over dive with a Navy F-14 next to a Russian MIG fighter.

One G force is the weight of gravity. It is not uncommon for a jet to pull 4 G's in the course of its maneuvers. The spine and body are compressed like sardines, then stretched out like rubberbands.

If you have ever watched the movies the late Art Scholl filmed in the cockpit of his jet during these maneuvers, you would see what I'm talking about. He had the camera pointed inside the cockpit, focusing on his face. You can see his skin grotesquely pushed and pulled away from the bones of his face as he does his dives and turns.

Think about the crew who works on the flight deck of aircraft carriers. They are constantly subject to lifting heavy tow mechanisms and equipment, exposed to jet exhaust and noise, and the constant stress of getting the planes and helicopters on and off the flight deck. Needless to say, chiropractors could have lots of work to do on an aircraft carrier!

Then there are all the other jobs in the military where men and women do heavy equipment work. Lifting, digging, laying wire, driving tanks and jeeps over rough terrain are just some examples. All of these jobs carry a risk of directly damaging the back.

There are also jobs which may compromise the person's health, such as people who work with dangerous chemicals or are under constant stress. These people could also benefit from the optimum health aspect resulting from chiropractic adjustments and the great reduction of stress after an adjustment.

Is it doing the military services any good if their people are laid up with painful backs? Instead, it would be beneficial to have commissioned doctors of chiropractic in the military to take care of personnel on a regular basis. Even the top generals and admirals may have back and health problems which can be helped with chiropractic care. If their health is maintained, I believe they would be better leaders. Everyone under their command would benefit, including the citizens of the United States who are dependent on our military forces for protection.

Once again, don't imagine that our work can be duplicated by an M.D. or physical therapist, unless of course they have also earned a doctor of chiropractic degree. Chiropractors are unique in their ability to balance and correct the spine. With our education we should be commissioned, and not be under the direction of the M.D., unless it is triage work in a MASH unit, where everyone's job is to help the surgeons. Since most medical doctors don't know what doctors of chiropractic do, how could they be competent to command us when it comes to administering our type of health care?

There is so much good that can be done and so much cost in terms of time and expense that can be saved by having commissioned doctors of chiropractic in the military. This is why relevant legislation was enacted. Unfortunately, despite the passage of the Senate bill, many medical military leaders are reluctant to cooperate. Many do not feel chiropractic can benefit the military, probably because they do not really know what we can offer. The bill has passed, and it is only a matter of time before chiropractors will be commissioned officers. I believe the M.D.s will then find their own job easier as they will not have to deal with soft tissue back injuries, except those serious cases requiring surgery.

9.   *Chiropractic and the Mentally Challenged:* There is a great deal about the body we do not understand. There is even more about the mind and the brain we don't understand. If we only use 2% – 3% of our mental potential, then why do such small lesions in the cerebral cortex cause such seemingly catastrophic events? Or if someone has a serious lesion of the brain and is labeled "brain damaged," how is it through positive reinforcement, training and lots of patience they can overcome the injury and lead a normal life?

Doctors and scientists can label mentally ill patients, but they cannot tell why they are disabled. They can use powerful drugs or electroshock therapy to control the symptoms, but they usually cannot stop the cause of the problem. In spite of all our knowledge, we really have only scratched the surface of the cause and correction of poor mental health.

Dr. B.J. Palmer, one of our founding fathers, said he would like to go into the mental houses of the nation and adjust all of the mentally ill. It was his belief that they all could be helped tremendously by the power of the chiropractic adjustment.

I have spoken of the work of Dr. Don Harrison of Alabama. In his analysis of how the atlas or C1 vertebra is positioned, Dr. Harrison has found one cause of mental illness. He and others who practice his technique of Biophysics take special x-ray views as developed in other techniques such as NUCCA and Toggle. These views show clearly how the atlas is positioned with respect to the occiput (skull) and the rest of the cervical spine.

Since 1986, I have heard hundreds of chiropractic miracle stories and have read many patient testimonials. I was working several years ago in Dr. Murphy's office when a new patient came in and told us about his condition. He said he had been diagnosed as a manic-depressive many years before, and he was coming in for relief from his severe headaches. He said everything started years before when he fell off a roof while working as a roofer. He said, "Now I get these headaches and they pound, and they POUND, and they POUND!

I was a student at the time and pretty green. I thought I was going to have to call someone for assistance because he was starting to whip himself into quite a lather. Dr. Murphy in his calm voice simply told him to say more about his case. The fellow quieted down somewhat and proceeded to tell us that his wife was leaving him, he couldn't work at his job any more, and that he was probably going to be committed.

Dr. Murphy took some x-rays of his upper cervical (neck) area and proceeded to adjust him. The man got up off the upper cervical table, looked around, smiled and said, "I feel great!" He proceeded to run around the office telling everyone how wonderful he felt, how everything was wonderful, and how chiropractors were the greatest doctors on earth. He started shaking Dr. Murphy's hand and wouldn't stop until Dr. Murphy slipped my hand into the man's grasp.

I then led the man out to his car (he was still pumping my hand up and down) and helped him into his front seat. I told him to come back in two days to be checked, finally got free of his hand, and said good-bye. To this day he still comes in for regular care and has not had any more episodes of manic depression. His life has been put completely back in order.

Allan G.J. Terrett reports that medical professionals Eric Milne, a general practitioner, and Frank Gorman, an ophthalmologist, studied several cases where patients with migraines, dizziness, depression, nervousness, irritability, disorientation, visual disorders, auditory difficulty, poor concentration, loss of interest in sex and several other problems were all helped by spinal manipulation. They proposed that the reduction of cerebral blood flow (blood to the brain) due to neck misalignment was not enough to kill the brain cells, but was enough to keep them from functioning. This loss of blood may not stop "core" brain functions such as eating, walking, or talking, but will affect the sophisticated brain functions.[76] These findings have been echoed in other cases where full visual loss has been restored by chiropractic adjusting, as well as the loss of speech and arm use.[77]

There are no limits to the benefits of good chiropractic care. We know of people who have done terrible things, people we have labeled crazy or dangerous, but we don't know the cause of their actions. Dr. Gerard Clum, President of Life Chiropractic College West, in a speech in October, 1994 related the story of Sirhan Sirhan, the assassin of Senator Robert Kennedy. He stated that Sirhan's mother had said Sirhan was never the same after a fall onto his neck from a horse. The mind can only guess at how this century might have been different if he had seen a chiropractor.

It may be true that many cases of mental illness are the result of other causes and may not respond as dramatically. However, it would still help the overall health of the patient to be adjusted. My advice would be to explain to the patient what is going on and get an examination by a competent chiropractor as soon as possible.

10. *Chiropractic and Animals—Bad Cases of Arfritis!*: People are often surprised when they go into their chiropractor's office and see someone's dog having its spine adjusted by the doctor. Cats, horses, dogs, sea mammals, lions, tigers (and bears, oh my!) have all received chiropractic care. In fact, any animal that has a spine may benefit from chiropractic care.

Chiropractic is about gaining and restoring health. It is possible that your pet may have had a fall, been kicked by a neighbor, or been in a fight and had one or more vertebrae knocked out of alignment which has caused swelling that compress or affect the nerves. Without treatment the animal may become sick and no one will know why. A veterinarian may find something wrong with the animal's organs, but may not relate the cause back to the spine. The vet may give drugs or operate on the organ which may control the symptoms. Just as with humans, if the cause of the trouble is at the spinal level, then the problem, if unresolved, may recur.

There are chiropractors in many areas who visit the horse racetrack early in the mornings and adjust the horses before they run. The owners and trainers have found their animals run faster, longer, and recover from training more quickly after a chiropractic adjustment. In many cases the chiropractors have conferred with veterinarians who have taught them the anatomy and physiology of the animals they are working on.

It is usually illegal for a chiropractor to work on an animal without a vet's approval. Veterinarians are interested in the animal's health, and there have been very few instances that I know of where the chiropractor has gotten into trouble with the law.

When I was a chiropractic student, my colleague and friend Dr. Darrell Lavin and I took a sports seminar from a chiropractor named George LeBeau, D.C. During the course of the class Dr. LeBeau told an unusual story and used a newspaper article to back it up.

Several years ago one of his patients, a police officer, told him about his dog. The animal was a German Shepherd used in the local K-9 unit on the police force. One day the dog was chasing a suspect. Just as the dog was about to catch up to him, the suspect turned and kicked the dog in the spine. Ever since then, the poor animal limped and could not run. Their vet tried everything, but could do very little. Subsequently the animal had to be retired from the police force.

When Dr. LeBeau heard this story, he asked if he could look at the dog. The owner readily agreed. Dr. LeBeau found the problem in the animal's spine: several vertebrae had been moved out of their normal position. This caused the spine to move improperly and probably caused the animal severe pain. After a few

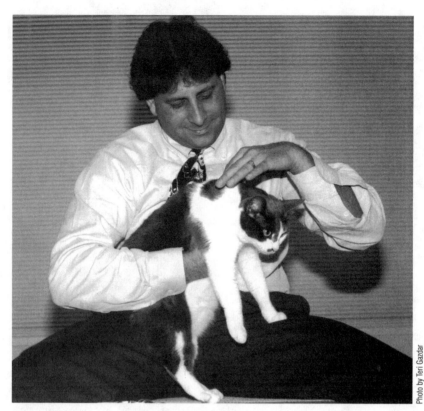

Photo by Teri Gazdar

Here the chiropractor is adjusting the spine of a very ferocious house kitty. Adjustments are very gentle.

adjustments, the dog began to improve rapidly. Eventually he healed completely and returned to the police force.

These stories are not uncommon; there are videos and books on how to adjust animals. The reaction from the animals is often strange. For example, I've had dogs turn around after I adjusted them and lick my hand, but sometimes when I adjust cats, they will leap off my lap straight up into the air and dash away!

One brief note. If your chiropractor agrees to adjust your pet, he or she may ask you to bring the animal in at the end of the day. Don't be insulted! Your chiropractor is a people doctor first and foremost and may not want the rest of the patients seeing animals in the clinic. The chiropractor may want a three-way consultation with you and the animal's veterinarian to discuss your pet's condition and to reassure the vet that you really desire this adjustment for your animal. This can be a good idea that may bring unexpected rewards, such as the vet and chiropractor working together on future cases.

8

Myths about Chiropractic

Health really does comes from within.

It is true that chiropractic has been a long time in coming and gaining acceptance. Times have definitely changed. My purpose here is to relate some of the myths and half-truths (or half-lies) that persist. You may have heard some of them and hopefully your mind is not closed to my point of view. Some of these tales will be new to you, and I hope you get a laugh out of them.

1. *"I don't believe in chiropractors."*

One of the funniest things I hear from prospective patients is that they would come see me but they don't believe in chiropractors, as though we were ghosts. I usually feign surprise and say, "Well, I'm really standing here. Touch my arm if you don't believe me!"

One fellow once told me he would never ever go to a chiropractor. He made back supports for a medical company and had heard stories from the medical orthopedist he worked for. I asked if he had ever been to a chiropractor, and he replied he never had and he never would. I asked if he knew anything about chiropractic, and he said that he didn't want to know anything. I asked if he had ever had the chance to observe what a chiropractor does, and he said no and he didn't want to observe one. In exasperation, I asked finally if he had ever talked to anyone who had been helped by a chiropractor, and he said he had but assumed they didn't know what they were talking about. Now this is a man with his mind made up!

I finally told him that most prejudice about a subject, person or profession stems from being uninformed. I would have loved to talk to him about chiropractic, but I didn't think it would do any good. I finally asked him if he had similar opinions about ethnic groups such as Blacks, Asians, or Hispanics. He didn't have an answer for that.

Chiropractic is not a religion. It is not just a philosophy, and it is not just a science. Like medicine, it is a philosophy backed up by science, and a science practiced with philosophy. It is not a question of believing in chiropractic or chiropractors, but whether or not you are open minded enough to try something different from traditional medical care; something that has been proven to be scientifically valid. It may take some courage on your part, but you have to make up your own mind that you have nothing to lose and everything to gain.

2.   *"Chiropractors will give you a stroke."*

This is one of the falsest statements and most misunderstood areas in chiropractic. Strokes are no laughing matter. I know of one prominent neurosurgeon (and there are several) who tells his patients never to go to a chiropractor because sooner or later chiropractors give their patients a stroke during a neck adjustment.

Let me say there is a possibility of this happening. With careful screening of patients and a thorough history and examination, the possibility of a stroke occurring is somewhere around 1 in 10 million adjustments, according to J. Cyriax, M.D.[78] Other estimates put it at 1 in 3.4 million—like being hit by lightening.

My question to that surgeon is how many patients has he operated upon who have developed strokes after his surgical procedure? The chance of suffering a stroke as a side effect is much higher for any surgical patient than for a chiropractic patient. Yet to the medical profession this is an acceptable risk, even for many elective operations. *(See chart)*

Some of the victims of spinal manipulation who have suffered stroke were already high-risk patients for strokes before they ever saw a chiropractor. People with a large amount of fatty plaque in their vertebral arteries are often candidates for strokes. Chiropractors are trained to do tests which help screen out these patients, but there is no guarantee of detecting all these conditions. What we try to do through these tests is lower the probability of an adverse reaction.

APPROXIMATE COMPLICATIONS OF MAJOR MEDICAL PROCEDURES PER ONE MILLION CASES:

Procedure	Complication	Rate per Million
1. Carotid entartectomy (surgery)	Stroke or Death	100, 000
2. Thoracic Aortic Aneurism (surgery)	Stroke	88,000
3. Coronary Artery Bypass Graft (surgery)	Stroke or Death	3,000 - 52,000
4. Use of Heparin & Streptokinase Therapy after a MI (heart attack)	Death	30,000
5. Neurosurgery for Neck Pain	Paralysis	15,000
6. General Anesthesia (complications from neck position)	Stroke or death	(Data Pending)
7. Use of Streptokinase Therapy without Heparin after a Myocardial Infarct	Death	8,000
8. Daily use of Aspirin to prevent Strokes & Heart Attacks	Stroke	7,000
9. Angioplasty (catheter balloon inserted into coronary artery)	Stroke	5,000
10. Unknown Causes of Strokes	Stroke	3,700
11. Chymopapain injections for Herniated Spinal Discs	Death	1,400
12. Chiropractic Cervical Adjusting	Stroke	1
13. Chiropractic Cervical Adjusting	Death	0.05

*Note: the above are approximations gleaned from various medical sources and special reports. This table is COPYRIGHT 1994, by W. Michael Gazdar, D.C. for use in his book: *Taking Your Back to the Future; How to have a pain-free back and total health with Chiropractic care.* Information compiled by W. Michael Gazdar, D.C. *(See References)*

There is a series of tests known as George's Test which is one way to screen patients. There are four parts to George's Test, including a history, blood pressure readings in both arms, listening for artery sounds known as bruits on both sides of the neck, and finally turning the head upward and to the right side and then to the left side, which causes a temporary decrease of blood flow to the brain. If any one of these tests is positive, given the parameters of the test, then rotatory (turning of the head to the side) cervical adjusting should not be done.

Another reason someone may have a stroke due to a cervical manipulation is if the adjustment is done too hard or not done by a doctor of chiropractic. Often people think they can do for others what their chiropractor has done for them. This is a mistake and may cost a life. I have watched people in gyms and weight rooms who may have been under chiropractic care at one time in their lives tell others that they know how to do manipulation of people's backs and neck.

I watched one fellow "adjust" a woman's neck by grabbing her chin with one hand, rotating her head as far to the right as he could, and with his other hand yanking on her neck as hard as he could. A loud snap was heard, along with the woman's yell of pain. Other than hurting her neck, I have always worried that she now believes that is how a doctor of chiropractic adjusts the neck. This is the Rambo style of "adjusting," not a chiropractor's!

Even some M.D.s who have attended weekend seminars on adjusting believe they are equal or superior to chiropractors in cervical adjusting. One case involved an M.D.'s cervical manipulation which caused a stroke in a 31 year old woman.[79] This article reviewed a case from December 1987 where the medical physician treated a woman for headache by using a cervical manipulation. This caused an immediate stroke due to the tearing of both vertebral arteries.

Some people might say no one should ever do a cervical manipulation because of the danger of stroke. This is like someone saying we should never do surgery or prescribe drugs or put people under anesthesia because there is a risk. The risk of stroke by cervical manipulation by a *properly* trained person is approximately

1 in 3.4 million. The physician mentioned in this article claimed to have taken a ten-week course at a chiropractic college and had a variety of chiropractic mentors who trained him, yet he was unable to produce either the mentors or the evidence that he had ever taken the course.

One of the plaintiff attorneys, Donald E. Karpel, Esq., said about the case, "I think it is a classic example of M.D.s who are unregulated by the medical profession and whose regulations allow these manipulations, in the face of some very severe red lights, causing our clients some very severe problems." He went on to say that, "I think this (incident) should really be publicized . . . . We should get the word out that (medical) doctors should stay in their realm. I think that chiropractic adjustments can be very beneficial to certain people where warranted…"

The implication here is that a trained chiropractor would have recognized that cervical manipulation for this particular patient would have been contraindicated in any circumstance and would not have performed an adjustment. Unfortunately, the M.D. did not have four years of chiropractic college behind him and did not recognize the warning signs.

On the subject of too forceful a manipulation, some practitioners are simply more heavy handed than others. If possible, you should inquire from current or former patients just how hard the doctor adjusts. This may save you searching from one doctor to another in order to find the right one. If cervical adjusting is a major concern to you, then seek out someone who practices "nonforce" techniques such as Activator, NUCCA or B.E.S.T. If you find you are not getting the relief you are looking for, then you may need to go to someone who moves the vertebrae somewhat more forcefully, but does not twist the neck. These techniques are Biophysics, Thompson-Pierce-Stillwagon, and other "Drop Table" techniques.

3.   *"Chiropractors make you come back to them forever."*

I have tried to demonstrate the need for care from the chiropractor's perspective. We would like you to be a patient for life, but this is your choice. If you have a desire to live a long, healthy and disease-free life, the probability of this improves with good, consistent care. As I have said before, it is similar to going to the dentist for a checkup twice a year. Chiropractic maintenance or prevention care tunes up your spine several times a year. Subluxations are simply "cavities" of the spine.

It's your body and you are the boss, regardless of what your doctor may tell you. If you follow the prescribed care, you should recover sufficiently. Normal prescribed care may vary depending on the severity of your health problem, so don't be surprised if you are seen daily or at least three times a week the first month, twice per week the second month or two, and once per week for the next two or three months. It takes time to retrain and reform the soft tissue around the vertebrae.

Many chiropractors will ask you if you want your problem corrected or if you just want symptomatic relief. Remember, the pain will usually go away long before the problem has been corrected. If you just want the quick fix, you do not have to worry about coming in forever, although the pain and the problem will probably recur. If you want correction, then you will want extended care.

Some people live their lives in a "crisis" type of mode. When their condition, weight, health or pain gets bad enough, they will get care until it goes away enough to provide relief. Then they move on to the next crisis. Other people like to prevent problems by watching their weight, taking vitamins, brushing their teeth and getting their spines checked regularly throughout their life. If you honestly state which type person you are, we chiropractors will understand the kind of care you want.

Some people respond slower and some respond faster. The chiropractor should be giving you periodic re-examinations every ten to twelve visits or so and checking with you to see what changes you are experiencing. The doctor's job is to tell you what you need, not just what you want to hear. If you disagree with his or her opinion, then speak frankly with them about it.

Once this "intensive period" is over and you are experiencing relief from your original condition, your spine should be in the correction or near-correction mode; maintenance or support care is recommended to insure that you avoid a relapse. It is as frustrating for the chiropractor as it is for the patient to have to go back and repeat all of the previous work because the condition was allowed to return.

For maintenance or support care your schedule may reduce to once or twice a month for a longer period of months or even years in order to prevent the problem from recurring. It varies from case to case. Both you and your doctor should know how long you are able to hold your adjustment before you slip out of alignment. Further, your chiropractor may elect to retake x-rays of the problem areas of your spine. This way he or she can evaluate how much spinal correction has taken place and how much more work is required.

4.   *"I went to a chiropractor once and it hurt more after than it did before, so I never went back."*

This is something I hear frequently. Think of how it would feel if you worked out hard in the gym and stretched muscles you hadn't stretched before. Wouldn't you expect to be sore? It is the same with a spinal adjustment. The chiropractor is stretching tissue that is not used to being stretched. The vertebrae, now in their correct position, are not accustomed to this new alignment and may be sore. The tissue of the facet joints in the back have been lengthened, and some of the adhesions which have been causing the problem have been broken. This is all good!

If you have ever had braces on your teeth, you know you go in to the orthodontist feeling fine, and after being adjusted usually feel sore the next day as the teeth adapt to their new position. It is the same concept with chiropractic adjustments.

On the other hand, if your symptoms have increased, the pain going down your leg or arm is worse, or you are feeling dizzy or nauseous, then you should call the chiropractor right away for a re-examination. He or she can determine if this is normal or if something is not right.

I always try to call my patients after the first adjustment to check in with them because I am truly concerned with their well being. Dr. Kirby Landis teaches this to all of his students, and it is something my patients always seem to appreciate. If the patient is experiencing some pain or discomfort, I can respond right away.

Often your chiropractor will tell you to apply ice or lie on certain blocks or pillows after the adjustment. This is to allow the body to rest and to heal better. Once the scar tissue has been disrupted, there might be a slight increase in discomfort as the body tries to handle this new "trauma." The ice decreases the swelling and does not allow the body to make as much new scar tissue. Lying on blocks and special pillows allows the tissues of the body to reform into new and better positions. All of this should help you to feel better, but if you consistently feel worse after the adjustment, you should call your chiropractor.

5.   *"Chiropractors think they can cure everything."*

By now you have some appreciation for the healing power of the body. Your body is truly an amazing machine, and you should respect and take care of it. However, if you have had some trauma or something didn't form correctly inside your body at some point in your evolution, then that is why God made doctors.

As I have explained in other parts of this book, we chiropractors do not do the curing. We simply remove nerve interference due to subluxations and let the body do all of the healing. Yes, we do believe the body can cure itself of almost anything given the right environment, but the doctor does not do the healing. Even the surgeon who repairs your heart is not responsible for the healing that takes place. It is the chiropractor's job to put the body into its optimum healing state so you can heal as quickly and completely as possible.

Think about the relationship of the nerves of the spine to the rest of the body's systems, including the muscle, skin and internal organs. By removing nerve interference or breaking the cycle of subluxation, the body will work more efficiently and naturally toward healing itself. If it can do this, it can avoid drugs, medications or invasive surgery.

The reason we need doctors other than chiropractors—such as allopaths, M.D. osteopaths, dentists, and others—is because the body cannot cure itself of everything. If you have had major trauma to the bones, skin, teeth, internal organs, vascular system, or you have been poisoned, you need to be seen medically. If you have had problems with the soft tissues and joints of the body and have not been able to get well with conservative chiropractic care, your chiropractor will probably send you to a medical specialist for a second opinion.

This is true of medical doctors as well, who send their difficult back cases to chiropractors for an opinion from a different perspective. Many M.D.s have told me that they don't understand the chiropractic philosophy of health, but they are willing to listen and make referrals if it will help their patients.

Sometimes we are misunderstood by the medical profession regarding the issue of healing. Dr. Grant A. Thompson, a chiropractor who has practiced over twenty years in Australia and is a friend of mine told me an interesting story. He was in the hospital to have a vein stripped from his leg.

The anesthesiologist was a cocky sort who didn't have a very high opinion of chiropractors. Just before he induced anesthesia, he asked Dr. Thompson who was going to watch his practice while he was in the hospital. Dr. Thompson said he had a partner who would take care of the patients while he recovered. The anesthesiologist said, "What's wrong, can't your partner fix the vein in your leg?" "No," replied Dr. Thompson, "and I'll tell you something else he doesn't do. He doesn't put a lot of people into the hospital with iatrogenic (doctor caused) disorders." And with that the anesthesiologist put him immediately to sleep!

6.   *"I don't need a chiropractor, I can "pop" my own back."*

Many people are reluctant to spend their hard earned dollars on anything other than the absolute necessities of life. Pleasures such as entertainment and good food are usually at the top of the list. Often health care is at the bottom of the priority list unless pain prevents you from doing the things you love or need to survive. Most chiropractors understand this. That is one of the reasons why chiropractic care is one of the least expensive ways to ensure your good health for many years to come. A small amount spent now is better than a large amount later. However, few things in life are free.

Many of my patients are people who have "popped" their own backs for years. They are also the ones who usually end up with the most severe problems. Even chiropractors cannot adjust their own backs, and we are the experts!

The joints of your back are designed to move a certain way and have a certain amount of elasticity. Your back should be able to stretch somewhat and then rebound to its normal position. Unfortunately, due to trauma, bad posture or extreme stretching on the part of the patient, the back may become restricted in motion. This is the "stuck-in-position" vertebrae or subluxation. Swelling results and the nervous system is adversely affected.

Other areas in the back will usually compensate for the subluxation by moving out of their normal position. These compensating vertebrae are usually easy to move back into place, while the subluxated vertebrae are harder to adjust. It is extremely difficult to lever your body into the proper position to adjust the correct joints.

When you grab your chin or your legs and twist your body to hear it pop, you are essentially wearing out the joints which are compensating for the subluxation instead of adjusting the subluxation itself. In other words, as you twist, all the compensating joints will stress and pop and the last to go will be the one(s) which are restricted. The stuck ones causing the problem may not move at all.

People who do this usually say they feel better, but the stiffness comes back fairly quickly. There is some reflex relaxation of the muscles, but usually the stiffness comes back within 20 to 60 minutes. You are making your overall condition worse as those areas become too loose or hypermobile. The subluxated vertebrae become more and more entrenched or hypomobile in their poor position. This increases damage to the nerves and joints involved. The compensated vertebrae that move are simply "the weakest link" in the chain and need to be left alone.

Chiropractors can locate the specific subluxated areas, adjust them, and leave the rest alone. Patients who have been able to "pop" their own backs report that after starting chiropractic care they are no longer able to self-adjust themselves. They also say they now feel much better and are free of pain. Their back is becoming healthier and the joints are not wearing out as fast.

As you continue to learn more about chiropractic care, you will probably hear more stories and myths about the chiropractic profession. Keep in mind we are a drug-less, non-surgical profession. Thus, we are often in competition with the American Medical Association and the pharmaceutical industry. These are powerful organizations who, some say, have manipulated the media and public opinion in the past. As an intelligent consumer, you have a right to the truth, not propaganda. That is one reason you are reading this book.

9

Chiropractic and Medicine—Sometimes the Combination can be a Healthy Mix

Take this magical pill and no matter what else you do to your body, you will be okay.

"Medical doctors love chiropractors, and chiropractors love medical doctors." Okay, this statement is not quite true yet, but some of us are working on it. For some practitioners just the opposite is true. Just as many races are still discriminated against in different areas of this country, it is still difficult for professionals to overcome their own forms of prejudice. Like the Berlin Wall, old barriers are being broken down every day, and out of the rubble new relationships are forming—with the patient's best interest in mind.

For chiropractors in particular, this is the most exciting time to practice. Many new scientific studies have proven that chiropractic works better and faster than medical care for musculoskeletal problems. Many pro-chiropractic medical articles are leading more and more people to turn to chiropractic care. Many medical doctors, frustrated by patients' complaints of constant back pain and poor health, are consulting with and referring patients to chiropractors.

A good friend of mine who is an orthopedic surgeon has often told me how frustrating it is for him to listen to patients complain about back pain and not be able to help them. He knows their problem is mechanical in nature, but not yet surgical. Medical doctors are grateful to have their patients get relief through chiropractic.

Patients will not think badly of the family physician who refers him to a trusted chiropractor to try and help. Instead they appreciate the doctor's attempt to find a cure rather than persist in applying different drugs with no results. They would respect their M.D. for admitting he or she cannot help the problem they are experiencing.

That was what I respected most about Dr. Paul Ryan, the medical doctor my mother worked for many years in Richmond, California. When Dr. Ryan didn't know something, he would tell the patient he wasn't sure what was going on and would either research the problem by going to the medical library or send the patient to a specialist. The chiropractor is a specialist of the spine and dis–eases which emanate from the spine. The chiropractic/medical mix is proving to be a good relationship, though still a tentative one, for all parties.

As mentioned in the beginning of this book, traditional bio-medical models are based on the reductionist theory. They try to break every disease and disorder down to the cellular level. This is good in many instances, but often inappropriate when dealing with people and their pain. Humans are complicated!

Irvin Korr, Ph.D. said you can study all the chemical characteristics of hydrogen and oxygen, but this tells you nothing about what they become when combined — water (H_2O). He says science ignores the individuality of patients and the reasons why disease occurs.

Chiropractic looks at the total health and lifestyle of the individual and tries to incorporate all aspects of that person's life. This has helped chiropractors get the reputation as "human doctors." This seems to have some influence on the medical community, as it is now looking at patients more as people rather than merely as disease entities.

Chiropractic and Other Health Disciplines

You probably have learned from the previous chapters that your chiropractor works with the entire body, which means that he or she could conceivably relate with any type of doctor. We will concentrate on just a few appropriate examples.

1.   *Podiatry:* The podiatrist specializes in the treatment of disorders of the feet. Podiatrists can be especially important to the chiropractor and to the chiropractic patient. The spine is the most important structure in the body because it houses the nervous system, but the spine is supported by the legs and the legs by the feet.

The feet have moveable joints just like the rest of the body. If the feet are misaligned, either through hammer toes, pinched nerves, or an imbalance of some sort, there will be torquing of the long bones of the legs in a compensatory way. This throws the pelvis out of alignment, which further causes subluxations and compensations all the way up the spine.

I had one patient who had severe headaches. We worked on his neck (often the source of bad headaches) and on his middle and lower back for other problems. We had some success with the headaches, but they didn't go away completely. As we began rehabilitating his ankle for an old sprain that had healed badly, his ankle began to respond to the adjustments and the physical therapy. We noticed that the ligaments held their corrected position longer and his headaches stopped altogether.

Many chiropractors prescribe foot orthotics to their patients in order to stabilize the feet and the spine. Anything we can do to get the adjustment to hold longer and decrease the frequency of visits to the chiropractor is desirable.

Sometimes it is necessary to have the patient's feet examined by a competent podiatrist prior to prescribing orthotics. A podiatrist may see the need to remove corns, bunions or other maladies of the feet before the cast is made. If these maladies are treated after the cast has been made and the orthotics fitted, the orthotics may not fit correctly after the treatments and will be of little use to the patient. The podiatrist will also do a very detailed examination of the feet and note if there are medical problems which must be addressed.

One thing a chiropractor may do that a podiatrist might not do is to adjust the bones of the feet in a similar way to spinal adjusting. This requires specialized training that chiropractors receive that most podiatrists do not get. Podiatrists who do have this specialized training become incredibly adept at foot manipulation. If you think you need this type of care, look in the Yellow Pages or ask for a referral to a chiropractor or podiatrist who specializes in sports or extremity adjusting.

2.   *Dentistry:* The biggest impact of the merger between dentistry and chiropractic is on the successful management of patients with Temporal Mandibular Joint ("TMJ") dysfunction. TMJ is a source of a great deal of suffering for many people. Anyone who has ever had direct trauma to the jaw, worn braces, broken a tooth while chewing hard food, experienced bite problems, or been in an auto accident is a possible candidate for TMJ problems.

The muscles which may contribute to the TMJ problem are the masseters, temporalis, and the pterygoids. These are all powerful muscles which are involved in chewing and in TMJ movement. These muscles may become spastic and cause clenching in addition to grinding of the teeth at night.

There is a small disc which lies between the mandible (lower jaw) and the maxilla (upper jaw) and acts as a cushion between them. If the mandible becomes jammed backwards, as with a direct blow, the disc may slip forward and displace. The muscle may spasm and continue the cycle of pain and grinding.

Dr. Dan Murphy has developed a technique for adjusting the jaw back into place using gentle traction. First he massages the spastic muscles of the side of the face such as the temporalis and masseters. Then he has the patient open his mouth, and he strokes the pterygoid muscles inside the mouth until they relax and release. Finally he has an assistant hold the patient's head while he gently tractions the jaw down and to the side. This creates enough of a space for the tiny disc to slip back to its normal position. It is generally painless and very effective.

Other chiropractic methods have developed their own unique way of adjusting the TMJ using Biophysics, Activator Methods, Gonstead and Diversified techniques among others. If you are curious about this subject, ask your doctor of chiropractic how he or she adjusts the TMJ and how well this has worked for them.

New information is also emerging which shows that problems with the TMJ are not just caused by problems with the joint, but also by cervical, thoracic, and even lumbar dysfunction. Teri K. Novak, D.C. was part of a team, including a dentist and a physical therapist, who presented a workshop called "Craniomandibular Dysfunction and TMJ Syndrome" at the American Back Society's Fall Symposium on Back Pain in December, 1990. The paper was reproduced in the *California Chiropractic Journal.*[80] In her paper, Dr. Novak cites several references which show why many dentists experience frustration in stabilizing patients with TMJ disorders who have postural faults and bad body mechanics. She also mentions whiplash injury as a cause of TMJ dysfunction, due in part to the splinting and spasm of critical muscles in the region, which in turn cause asymmetrical forces on the jaw.

3.   *Physical Therapists:* Sometimes there is a bit of animosity between chiropractors and physical therapists. This is unfortunate and possibly stems from the "turf battles" I have spoken of earlier. In my opinion, good physical therapists are worth their weight in gold.

When working with a post-trauma patient, I make sure the spine is aligned and the joints are in order, but sometimes I prefer to leave the rehabilitation of the tissues (stretching, strengthening, walking, work-hardening exercises) to physical therapists. They do a phenomenal job with these patients.

Even though I am the treating physician and like to be kept informed of what is being done, the therapist should have as much latitude as needed in order to accomplish what needs to be accomplished. With this "team approach" to patient care, everyone wins.

I would never let a physical therapist adjust the spine of my patient, and some chiropractors choose not to do physiotherapy modalities (high volt galvanic, diathermy, or ultrasound) in their office. Chiropractors are trained to use these modalities, and some reason that it is less expensive for the patient to get this care in their office while receiving an adjustment.

Some physical therapists do not like the fact that chiropractors use these modalities. According to Donald Dee Wesdorf,

D.C., a law in California dating back to 1922, and recently upheld, allows the chiropractor to perform physiotherapy modalities on patients in the office. Dr. Wesdorf has been a chiropractor for many years and says that chiropractors were among the early pioneers to make physical therapy modalities popular in the treatment of soft tissue injuries. The chiropractor does have the right to put his training to use.

If the patient is seeing a chiropractor, it may be more cost effective to do an ultrasound therapy in the chiropractor's office for an extra $20 (approximately) than to send them across town to the physical therapist's office where they may be charged $90 or more for an additional office visit. My objection is when the patient needs the services of a physical therapist, not just the modalities, and the chiropractor refuses to refer him or her to a physical therapist. Some therapists do adjust the patient's spine, although most are not trained nor qualified to do this. Indeed, in some states it is illegal.

Another difference between chiropractors and physical therapists is that chiropractors are considered primary care providers, along with medical doctors, osteopaths, podiatrists, dentists, and optometrists. This means that you do not need a referral from anyone to be examined and treated. A primary care provider is trained in diagnostic procedures related to that specialty and will treat you according to protocol. Physical therapists may in some states see a patient without a referral from a doctor. They are highly trained and experts in their field, but for the most part they work for and with the referring primary care provider.

If you sprain your ankle, either the chiropractor or the physical therapist can rehabilitate the local tissue for you. However, the chiropractor will also check and analyze your spine. This is because there are spinal segments known as neuromeres which correspond to the different regions in the body. There is a particular neuromere which corresponds to that ankle. The chiropractor will adjust that spinal segment, relieve the pressure on the nerves (subluxation) if there is one, and effectively speed up the healing of the ankle. In this way, chiropractors will always be an important part of sports medicine, along with the physical therapists.

Nutrition and Back Health

You truly are what you eat! Whatever you put in your body goes to your cells as food. Consider your body to be a Rolls Royce automobile. Would you put sugar into your gas tank the first thing in the morning before you drive? Of course not. Why would you purposely destroy your internal engine with highly refined sugars, drugs, alcohol or cigarettes?

Fatty foods followed by too many proteins may allow the body to build up antibodies to the proteins. This may be the cause of many auto-immune diseases such as Systemic Lupus Erythematosus (SLE) or Rheumatoid Arthritis (R.A.).[81] Fats slow down digestion so it takes twice as long to digest your food. The proteins sit for long periods of time waiting for digestion. Eventually the body may begin to develop an adverse reaction to the proteins, as it does to other foreign substances in the body. Thus, the body may begin to attack the proteins.

The tissues of your body are made up of these same proteins. The body is unable to distinguish the good proteins which make up your body from the proteins it has begun to fight. This may be the basis for many of these types of auto-immune diseases.

Many Americans are vastly overweight. This is not only due to lack of exercise, but also to eating high concentrations of fried, fatty foods, along with sugar and alcohol. High concentrations of "garbage" foods not only lead to being overweight but, according to John Robbins in his fine text *Diet For a New America,*[82] may also be responsible for an increase in cancer, colon irritation and diabetes.

This opinion is also expressed by John A. McDougall, M.D., in his book *McDougall's Medicine: A Challenging Second Opinion*[83] who points out that women in societies where the principal diet is starch, and where very few fats or animal products are eaten, have much lower rates of breast cancer. Excess estrogen, which is normally excreted by the colon, is reabsorbed back into the bloodstream in the presence of fats. Women whose diet is centered around starches and fiber have very little excess estrogen reabsorbed. The excess estrogen over stimulates certain kinds of hormone-responsive tissues in the breast and may be the mechanism which causes the tumor to form.

I recommend a balanced diet, low in fat and proteins and high in complex carbohydrates. If you are doing serious athletic training, you may wish to increase your intake of proteins slightly.   I also recommend dietary supplements of the vitamins C, A, and E. A good multi-vitamin with balanced multi-minerals should be taken as well. All vitamins should be time-released so as not to overload your body at one time. Vitamins A, E, and K are fat–soluble, which means they accumulate in the fat of your body. Accumulation may be harmful, and for this reason you may consider taking them for three or four days, then skipping a day. Any questions you have may be answered by your doctor or a nutritionist.

In *Confessions of a Medical Heretic*, Robert S. Mendelsohn, M.D. takes a swipe at modern medicine. He says that in every other system of medicine in the world there is a heavy emphasis on food for therapy, except for medical practice in the Western world. He feels that modern medicine has substituted drugs for food. Most American doctors completely disregard this nutrition except for certain "therapeutic diets" when treating diabetes, gout, hypertension or high cholesterol. Unfortunately, their approach is fragmentary and usually based on incorrect principles. He goes on to show how important nutrition is in oriental medicine, even to the person's spiritual well-being.

Chiropractic and the Insurance Game

Who is in control here?

At the time of this writing most insurance companies cover chiropractic care in whole or in part. Many have restrictions, just as they do in medicine, concerning the type of treatment, condition, and number of visits allowed. The difference is that most insurance before the 1990's was known as indemnity insurance. This means that you chose your doctor, submitted your bills, and either you or your doctor were reimbursed according to a percentage and after your deductible was met.

Now most insurers have moved away from this system in favor of Preferred Provider Organizations (PPOs) and Health Maintenance Organizations (HMOs). These are much more complicated. You will not always get your choice of doctor, and you may have to wait longer to see your physician. If you are in a HMO, you will have to go through a "gatekeeper," usually an M.D. who has a family practice, before you are referred out for any specialty. You need to know that in most cases family practice physicians are actively discouraged from making these referrals.

Even many insurance companies who were previously indemnity carriers are now contracting with HMOs and PPOs because they have been promised reduced claims. The HMOs and PPOs do this by denying care to you, the insured, and by denying payment to the doctors. What has happened is they have introduced more "middle men" who take their cut of the profits while driving up the cost and driving down the quality of health care.

You should know that some insurance companies are dropping chiropractic care because they say it is too costly. They are just trying to cut the excess. It may surprise you to know that out of over $900 billion spent on health care (actually disease care) in the United States in 1993, less than $4 billion was spent on chiropractic care. That is less than 0.5% of the total budget. Now where is the excess?

When the Manga Report came out of Canada, it proved the Canadian government could save $70 million per year by using chiropractors instead of medical doctors as the portal of entry—as primary care givers for back problems.[84] As the United States has 10 times as many people as Canada, this would translate into a $700 million savings per year! One wonders why there has not been greater coverage of this issue in the United States media.

DOONESBURY   **By G B Trudeau**

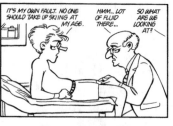
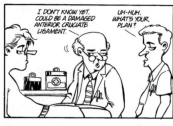
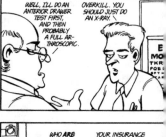
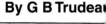
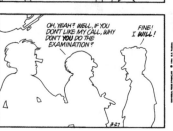
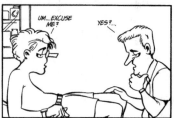
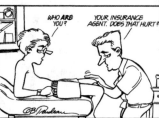

Courtesy of United Press Syndicate, used by permission.

1.   *Workers' Compensation and Personal Injury* I am most familiar with California laws since that is where I practice. Most states, including California, have favorable industrial and personal injury provisions so that chiropractic care for on the job injuries and auto accidents are covered at 100%. Many people are not aware that they may go to a chiropractor of their choice if they are

hurt on the job or injured in an automobile accident. Further, they are seldom told by their employer that they may predesignate a personal chiropractor or a personal physician, even though the current laws say employers must allow this. Unless these prior arrangements are made, an employer has the option of sending a worker to the company doctor for evaluation and care for the first 30-360 days (depending on the policy) following the on-the-job accident. After that period the worker may request a change of doctor if necessary or desired.

There is good reason for chiropractic care to be instituted in the workplace. A recent study showed that chiropractic care for workers' compensation cases in Utah was significantly less expensive than medical doctors' counterparts. The study examined 3,062 workers' compensation cases which occurred in Utah in 1986. Excluding surgical cases, the study revealed the average chiropractic patient lost only three days on the job compared to the physician patients who lost almost 21 days.

In addition, the average compensation was higher for the physicians: $684 compared to $527 for the chiropractors. The chiropractic patients received over two and one half times as many treatments on average as the physician patients, but the cost was less per visit and less overall.[85]

Other studies have echoed these findings.[86] All prove chiropractic to be the most efficient, lowest cost and the most satisfying to the patient of any medical alternatives available for musculoskeletal disorders.

Since chiropractors are now being recognized as the experts on musculoskeletal trauma that occurs on the job, whether lifting or sitting, many are being invited into the workplace to share their knowledge. For example, Scott Donkin, D.C., author of *Sitting on the Job*,[87] gives lectures on ergonomics and personally goes into offices to evaluate the worker's posture and job habits. He then offers recommendations on how to retrofit existing furniture and how to select new furniture which can help prevent on-the-job injuries. His book is a must for anyone who sits for long periods of time at a desk. Many other chiropractors, including myself, have taken Dr. Donkin's training and offer this health and cost saving benefit to employers.

Another pioneer chiropractor is Dr. Theodore Oslay, who focuses more on industrial workers. He will go into a facility, evaluate the work conditions, make recommendations on fixing problems which exist, and even set up a program of care that is relatively inexpensive and focuses on prevention. His staff will rehabilitate and treat workers on the job site and, if more extensive care is needed, will take the workers to a properly trained chiropractor in the area. He has cut the need for carpal tunnel and low back surgeries from thirty or more per year down to zero per year and has personally saved companies thousands of dollars. If that isn't cost cutting/life-changing work, I don't know what is!

Many personal injury cases, such as whiplash from automobile accidents, are also musculoskeletal in nature. Here again, chiropractors are now finally being considered the experts in the care and rehabilitation of soft tissue injuries. When your neck and/or low back is whiplashed in an auto or some other type of vehicle accident, there will probably be damage to the soft tissue of the spine, namely the ligaments, tendons, and muscles. The direct result of this is swelling, and the damaged tissue will be replaced by tough fibrotic tissue (scar tissue).

Many insurance adjusters will try to tell you that all you need is six to eight weeks of care and you will be fine. What they fail to tell you, whether out of lack of knowledge or because they want you to sign a quick settlement, is that tissue regeneration takes six to eight weeks, but tissue remodeling takes up to a year or longer.

Without extended chiropractic care you will heal, but your tissue will not heal properly and you will always have some pain. The tissue will become hypersensitive to any pressure or pain. There is a name for this: denervation supersensitivity. It is the reason for chronic pain after an accident. The victim's nervous system has changed and the pain threshold has lowered.

It has been found that continued chiropractic care after an accident results in a lower frequency of chronic pain. It may take several months following an accident for the full effects of the soft tissue damage to be felt. A person may feel fine at first, and as the tissue swells and changes, the pain starts to be felt. For this reason many chiropractors recommend you do not close a personal injury case for at least one year following the trauma.

An important part of your settlement should be for future care on an "as needed" basis. This is called future management or support for palliative purposes (flare-ups) in times of increased use and/or stress. It is hard to predict, but your chiropractor can often give you a reasonably good estimate depending on the severity of your condition. It is the job of the insurance carrier to return you to pre–injury status, or get you to maximum medical improvement, not fix every back problem you had prior to the accident. Patients, doctors and insurance carriers must be fair and reasonable at all times.

2.   *Medicare.*   Medicare can be a Nightmare. There are stiff penalties if the doctor does anything unacceptable with the billing. Many doctors are stuck with the dilemma of refusing the elderly who really need the care, or going along with the system and either not getting paid enough to cover office paperwork and the time it takes to process the forms and/or worrying that some innocent mistake made on billing is going to cost thousands of dollars in penalties per incident! These fines can be levied without any due process of law. This is why some doctors have stopped treating Medicare recipients unless they pay cash, which is unfortunate.

Some people have Medicare in addition to their other medical insurance. Often this helps them afford better care. They are able to submit their bills to both sources and have far lower co-payments.

Some companies are emerging which agree to take care of all of the complicated paperwork while receiving care in exchange for turning over your Medicare benefits to them. You should know that you may lose some services in this type of system. You may have to see their doctor at their frequency or even lose the chiropractic benefits which are part of Medicare.

The chiropractic benefits under Medicare are not that great. Currently you are entitled to only twelve visits per year, which is probably not enough in most cases. X-rays are required every year but not paid for by Medicare. Thus, they force you to have a procedure, but refuse to pay for it. The system needs to be revised.

3. *Personal Insurance*

Personal insurance may see a radical change in the next few years with a trend towards socialized medicine. The Clinton Administration tried its best to bring health care costs down. However, more government control may not be the best solution. For the citizen's sake it is logical that chiropractic care be included in a national health plan, but there is no guarantee.

Chiropractic is becoming the fastest growing health care system in America. In a 1991 meeting of the North American Spine Society, chiropractic treatment (a/k/a spinal manipulation) received very high ratings by the researchers. *Spine* is one of the most respected and prestigious journals concerning disorders of the spine. The experts on the panel were all medical doctors.

They included chiropractic care under the heading "Manual Therapy" and outlined what they thought was clinically acceptable for treating disorders of the lumbosacral spine.[88] The importance of this is that chiropractic should be included in any type of national health care system. Even if chiropractic is not included in a future national health policy, it should be noted that chiropractors have always been busy because people want and need the care.[89]

For example, during the Depression of the 1930s, many people were sick and out of work. The chiropractors of that era say they were busier than ever because people had to work but could not because of back pain and poor health, so they went to their chiropractors. Of course, during this time people could not always pay their chiropractic doctors with money. Some paid with chickens, eggs, meat, milk, or other commodities, but the people went to doctors of chiropractic in droves. This is further testimony to the importance of chiropractic care.

Currently, chiropractic is the second largest health care system in the world behind medicine and the largest natural, alternative care system. In 1993, citizens of the United States spent over $50 billion out of their own pockets for alternative health care. The government needs to wake up! People are searching for a new model for health, and chiropractic is redefining health and what constitutes a way back to recovery.

Economically, it would be beneficial if people were allowed chiropractic care, but it will take a lot of lobbying and public demand to get it passed into law. If you want to be guaranteed chiropractic care and get decent benefits, lobby your congressmen and senators. Tell them of the Manga Report from Canada. The researchers proved that chiropractic care was not only safer and more effective than medicine for back pain, but the Canadian government would eventually save BILLIONS of dollars if the management of low back pain were transferred to chiropractors.

Since the United States has a larger population than Canada, those savings would translate into even larger figures here. Nothing sways politicians' minds like public opinion. Tell them you do not want ridiculous limitations on your care if you are injured or suffer from a bad back or poor health. You have to DEMAND it!

Some insurance companies are better than others. Whenever you are considering a health plan, you should inquire whether or not the plan covers chiropractic care and what are the limitations of the plan. Some health plans cover up to a dozen visits per year, which may be realistic if you are only on maintenance care, but is totally inadequate if you are having almost any kind of an acute or subacute back problem.

For example, there is the concept mentioned above known as remodeling which involves the small intrinsic muscles of the spine. As the joint is restricted in its motion, i.e., subluxated, the muscles on one side become chronically stretched, weaker and remodel themselves accordingly. At the same time, the shortened muscles actually remodel themselves to stay shortened. When the chiropractic thrust is forced into the locked facet, the motion is restored. This is exactly what is supposed to happen, but since there has been remodeling, the joint will probably lock up again. It may take several months of care to for the muscles to remodel back to their proper lengths.

In addition to restricted access to the chiropractor, insurance policies often have a $250 deductible per year and allow $20 per session for up to twelve visits. Then they send you a letter saying the entire amount has been applied to your deductible and they are sending no money. Now you are stuck with the doctor's bill. Great policy!!

They may give the provider a fee schedule. When your doctor bills according to that schedule, they cut the charges, claiming fees are too high. These are other ways of not paying their fair share, but they always make sure to collect your premiums!

Many visit restrictions apply only to doctors of chiropractic and not to any other health provider. This is illegal and violates antitrust laws. An insurance company is required to pay for the service rendered, regardless of the type of doctor who performs it (as long as the doctor is licensed to perform the procedure). This is especially important when chiropractic has proven to be more successful than medicine in helping musculoskeletal problems.

On the other hand, there are insurance companies which do pay for chiropractic services in the same way as they pay medical doctors, podiatrists, physical therapists, or any other provider. Some have unlimited coverage and reasonable limitations. Most chiropractors don't expect carte blanche when it comes to health insurance, but a reasonable amount of coverage should be given, at least enough to cover the acute, subacute and chronic phases of an injury.

When patients are thinking about changing or choosing an insurance company, you can bet I will share my opinion on which ones are the best and which ones they should avoid. The best person to pressure if you want good, fair chiropractic benefits is your insurance representative.

As mentioned above, many chiropractors have begun to establish some sort of standards of care for the industry, including the types of care given, the number of visits per case, and a chiropractic regulatory board made up of chiropractors to enforce the committee rules. This was developed at the Mercy Conference, which took place in January of 1992, at the Mercy Center Hospital in San

Francisco. The guidelines have been published and they are being tested and reviewed, although many states have rejected them.

A few states have adopted the Mercy guidelines, but most have not. Many chiropractors fear that how to care for their patients will be dictated to them, but it is possible to have workable standards of care even if they only loosely bind the chiropractor. There already is an established code of ethics we all follow.

Some chiropractic techniques encourage re-x-raying the problem area after you have been under care for awhile. Biophysics, for example, is based on the premise of correcting bad posture, and it is relatively easy to show progress. As the patient improves, the spinal changes are demonstrable on film and can be correlated. Some critics claim this is too much radiation exposure, and in some cases it may be unless you are only getting one or two "spot shots" of the problem area.

Both you and the doctor will definitely know when you are fixed. If you simply wait for your symptoms to go away and then drop out of care, this is usually too soon. If your doctor has kept you around for several years at a high frequency of adjustments (such as eight to twelve visits per month) and has never told you what you are working toward, you may want to find out. You need both a goal and a plan when to stop active care and go on to support care (usually once or twice per month). Insurance companies are much more cooperative about paying if they know you are getting better and not just staying around to pad the bill.

One final thing to consider when purchasing health insurance: find out if your policy can be cancelled or restricted in the future if you make any claims against it. This is another unfair practice which could be financially devastating for the patient. Many AIDS and cancer patients and their families have been financially ruined by this practice as the insurance stops paying as the disease progresses.

Be careful with pre-existing condition clauses to your policy. If you have been under care for back problems, they may restrict your access to a chiropractor or other back specialists.

As the consumer, you do have a choice when it comes to purchasing health care coverage. Stand up for your rights to see not only the type of doctor you want, but also the individual doctor of your choice. It is your body and you are paying good money to insure it. If the insurance company wants you to see their particular doctor, ask if you can see your personal doctor instead. Tell them you will pay the difference between what your doctor charges and what their doctor charges (many insurance companies will agree to do this). If they don't let you do this, find one that will.   Whatever you do, don't let them bully you. Insurance is BIG business. It is no secret that some of the largest buildings in the world belong to insurance companies. If enough people demand fair health care, it will happen. Make sure adequate chiropractic care is included!

4.   *Chiropractic and Life Insurance*

It would be very profitable to life insurance companies if they only insured healthy people or those who don't pursue activities that may cause them harm. No one can look into a crystal ball and tell someone how healthy they will be or how long they will live. In many cases however, diseases are the result of a lifetime of abuse to the body.

If we are all surrounded by pollens and toxins in foods and the atmosphere, why are only some of us adversely affected? It's because of our immune systems. A good guideline for insurance companies would be a thorough examination of the person's immune system, for it is there that health is really determined. How does one do this? In a typical insurance examination, an applicant's blood pressure, pulse, and respiration rates are determined; routine lab tests are performed and sometimes an electrocardiogram (EKG) is given to check the heart. In addition to a health history, these measures are used to determine if the person is a good risk for the company.

These tests are fine for determining the individual's state of health at that time and may contain some future indications, yet what is sadly lacking in most cases is a thorough spinal assessment. The spinal exam can help to predict future medical problems better and quicker than many other tests. A direct cor-

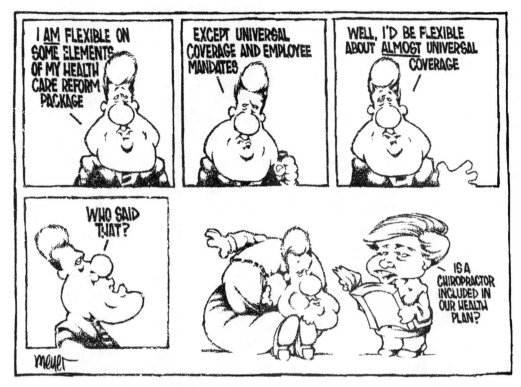

Courtesy of the San Francisco Chronicle, used by permission.

relation can be made between the spine and the immune system. No one is more qualified to perform this than a chiropractor.

Chiropractic works with the nervous system, which directly controls the immune system.[90] With vertebrae misaligned or abnormal posture, the nerves in that area do not function correctly and their corresponding organs will be adversely affected. It may soon be that one requirement for obtaining term life insurance is that you, the patient, are under some kind of spinal care, preferably chiropractic.

Chiropractors are in the business of keeping your nervous system intact and functioning as close to 100% efficiency as possible. We want you to live a long time despite what you do to your body.

Perhaps you've heard this tale: Once upon a time an elderly couple passed away within one month of each other. Since the wife preceded her husband, she was waiting for him along with St. Peter at the Pearly Gates. They greeted him warmly and took him on a tour of heaven. St. Peter proudly pointed out the beautiful golf courses, all with no waiting, the beautiful waterfalls and gardens, the wonderful banquet facilities available any time, day or night, the unlimited bowling lanes and pool tables—all first class.

"In fact," said St. Peter, "anything a man could want can be found here."

The husband looked very glum.

"What's wrong, dear," the wife asked, "aren't you happy to be here?"

"Yes," said the elderly gentleman, "But I could have been here 20 years ago if it wasn't for that damn oat bran cereal and chiropractor you made me go to!"

Oh well, we can't please everybody!

People are living longer, healthier lives. By now you have a better understanding of how the nervous system works and how increasing the blood flow through the organs, stimulated by a healthy nervous system, will make you feel better and possibly live longer.

It may be that clinical trials are truly evidence, but I do not know one chiropractor who omits getting their spine adjusted regularly. Most chiropractors know that a healthy nervous system will keep them living longer and better. You can bet they also want their loved ones and patients to experience this. Of course, it is true your beneficiaries will have to wait longer to collect your life insurance benefits, but that's okay, isn't it? Why not let your great-great-grandchildren inherit your life insurance?

Chiropractic and the World

I had the opportunity to travel to Japan in 1991, and teach chiropractic at the Tokyo Chiropractic College and to the Japanese Chiropractic Society. I was a guest of the Dean of Life Chiropractic College West, Dr. Michael Schmidt. We taught for seven days and loved every minute of it.

Two things became apparent to me while we were there. First, almost everyone could benefit from chiropractic care. Many of the people we saw had terrible back problems. Quite a few were stooped over or walked with a pronounced lean to one side, and most of them weren't that old.

Second, chiropractic in Japan, as in the rest of the world, is vastly underutilized. These people need care and, they don't know where to turn. We found they have many misconceptions about chiropractic care. In Japan, many believe that chiropractors work on stiff shoulders and low back pain.

Much of this is promoted by heavy advertising from the medical community and drug companies in Japan. The people are inundated by constant advertising that promises drugs will take away the pain and cure the problem. It is true that the pain will probably be lessened with the drugs for awhile, but the problem will go untreated and in time will worsen.

When you begin to examine the state of the world's health, it becomes apparent that something needs to be done. The world needs a new model for health; perhaps chiropractic is the answer, or at the very least, part of the answer.

A positive first step is education for the patient. Part of our training mission in Japan focused on patient education and how to attract new patients to chiropractic care. Usually, if the patient has had good care with a chiropractor, he or she will refer family and friends.

Even more importantly, if a patient has been educated properly, they will become a chiropractic patient for life, coming in as needed for monthly or bi-monthly tune-up adjustments that contribute to a long and healthy life. Since much of what a chiropractor can offer is preventive care, many people are checked and adjusted before they have any problems. These people seem to get fewer colds and flu, and suffer less from allergies than people not under care.

Japan notwithstanding, most of the world is unaware of the role chiropractic can play in the individual's health. Many chiropractors are joining sports organizations such as Federation Internationale de Chiropratique Sportive (FICS), and travel all over the world to deliver care to athletes at sporting events.

Some chiropractors also participate in non-sport organizations that send them to deliver care to foreign indigenous populations. The results are usually the same: the people love the care. This is not just because it makes them feel better, but because many people, including those who are in more rural areas, are aware that they need this kind of care. They would trust their family's health to someone who uses their hands to heal naturally rather than drugs.

A friend of mine, Dr. Ron Fritz, who now practices in San Diego, California was working in the office of Dr. Ron Benson in San Jose, California a few years ago. Dr. Fritz told me many of the patients who received excellent care from Dr. Benson were migrant farm workers from Mexico. They needed the adjustments in order to work and earn food for their families. They would say, "We come to the doctors who use their hands to heal, not to those who give the drugs."

Another friend of mine, Doug Green, D.C., who travels with FICS and was the team physician for the Spanish Team in the 1992 Olympic Games in Barcelona, recently returned from doing chiropractic work in South America. He told me that everywhere he went people wanted to know about chiropractic care. He said he was treated like royalty, even by the medical and military establishments. Like many others, he feels the world is wide open and ready to experience what chiropractic has to offer.

In many countries medicine has fallen short in all but the most life-threatening cases, and people want a change. Even though there are not very many chiropractic colleges outside the United States, there will probably be many more developed around the world in the next few decades.

If you have any aspirations of becoming a chiropractor, please contact your local library, college or high school career center and get information about chiropractic. You may want to contact one of the chiropractic colleges directly, or you can contact me. My number can be found at the back of the book. If you decide to become a chiropractor and go to Life Chiropractic College West, I will probably be one of your instructors. See you there!

Afterward

Congratulations! Either you made it all the way through the book, or you are one of those delightful people who likes to read the back of the book first. In any event, I hope you have enjoyed the presentation up to now and have told your friends what you have learned about chiropractic. Undoubtedly, I have enlightened some of you on the wonders of chiropractic and its relationship to good and poor health.

Possibly, my views and opinions have made some of you angry because they may be radically different from your own. This may be especially true if you are in the medical area of the health profession. You may have your mind made up about how things should be; then again, I hope you are ready for a change.

If there is anything our present health care system does not seem to address, it is HEALTH. We seem to be excellent at replacing one bad habit with another, killing our bodies with toxins from food, air and water, and finally killing our minds with television and news trash.

Then, when we turn to our doctors, they can never really give us any effective solution unless it comes in the form of a pill, powder, potion or an emergency life-saving operation. In most cases, this simply adds to the poison level of our bodies, and further taxes an already overburdened liver and immune system.

Please understand, I have not purposely tried to anger anyone; instead I've tried to present a different perspective and different model for health. I want you to be healthy! My opinion and my challenge to you is this: if health really comes from inside the body, and I believe it does, then what is the solution to all this Dis–ease?

Chiropractic may not be the whole answer, but it is definitely a large part of the solution. Think of the things you have learned. You can benefit immediately from your new knowledge about your health. If you are now seeing a chiropractor, you are beginning to enjoy the benefits of a healthier spine and ultimately, a healthier body.

If you are not seeing a chiropractor and you have a health concern, get checked as soon as possible. There are many good doctors of chiropractic out there; you just have to find them. I will be more than happy to assist you in any way. I appreciate your reading this book and would be proud if you would consider me to be your friend. I encourage you to get in touch with me if you have a health question, if you are trying to find a chiropractor, or just to tell me how you are doing. My number is listed at the end of this section.

I would also hope you are now stimulated to do some further research on your own, preferably constructive reading which would show new and better techniques for taking care of people. That is really what this is all about, not sacrificing one system of health care for another.

One final thought: If you are considering trying chiropractic for the first time, obtain a referral from someone you trust and just do it. Don't listen to negative advice from anyone. Make up your own mind. Don't let anyone rob you of your right to good health! And remember:

THE WORLD IS GETTING ADDICTED
TO FEELING HEALTHY!!
W.M.G. 1990-1997

Send correspondence/book orders to:

W. Michael Gazdar, D.C., C.C.S.P.
John Muir Chiropractic Center
1776 Ygnacio Valley Road
Suite 201
Walnut Creek, CA 94598

(925) 939-1738

Quantity discounts available

Glossary

Annular Rings: The fibrous outer portion of the intervertebral disc.

Anomaly: A congenital defect in the structure of the spine.

Cavitation: When a synovial joint opens up under pressure, causing an expansion of gasses and a decrease of tension in the joint; similar to removing a champagne cork. When done by a chiropractor to a tight joint, there will be an immediate increase in the range of motion.

Cervical: Uppermost seven vertebrae supporting the head.

Chiropractic: A system of therapeutics that attributes disease to dysfunction of the nervous system and attempts to restore normal function by manipulation and treatment of the body structures, especially those of the vertebral column.[91]

Chiropractic Adjustment: Similar to cavitation, but in addition to a reduction in joint tension, there is also a corresponding change in adverse nerve function. This is where the greatest amount of emphasis is placed among practitioners.

Chiropractor: A person skilled in the practice of chiropractic and who has completed the required curriculum for the title Doctor of Chiropractic. The chiropractor manipulates or "adjusts" the vertebrae back to their normal, most functional spinal position, thus effecting relief of joint and nerve pressure.

Coccyx: Four to five tiny fused bones below the sacrum.

Disc: A flat pad of fibrocartilage between two vertebrae.

Facet: Small flat plane surface on the vertebrae which makes up part of the vertebral joint.

Herniated Disc: Also known as slipped or ruptured disc. When the nucleus pulposus leaks under pressure through the outer rings of the disc and bulges back toward the nerve or nerve root.

Intervertebral Foramina: The hole at the side of two vertebrae which joins together to form a joint. The nerve passes through this hole on each side.

Joint Manipulation: Primarily done by medical doctors, osteopaths and physical therapists. Joint manipulation is done with the emphasis on better joint mobility rather than a beneficial change in adverse nerve function. (The chiropractic term is "adjustment").

Kyphosis: The curvature of the thoracic and sacral spines in a backwards direction.

Ligament: Connective tissue which attaches bone to bone or cartilage to cartilage.

Lordosis: The curvature of the cervical and lumbar spines in a forward direction.

Lumbar: The five low back vertebrae which support the trunk and lower organs, including those used for digestion.

Nucleus Pulposus: Thick fluid center of the intervertebral disc.

Plexus: A network of nerves.

Sacrum: Five fused vertebrae in a triangular shape at the back base of the pelvis which are below the lumbars. Acts to support and stabilize the lumbars and pelvis during walking, sitting, and other low back uses.

Scar Tissue: Fibrotic, tough tissue which replaces soft, pliable tissue after some sort of trauma.

Scoliosis: Curvature of the spine in a lateral direction.

Spine: The bony structure which houses the central nervous system. It is made up of a series of moveable bones called vertebrae.

Subluxation: Early 1900's; A subluxation is when one or more vertebrae has moved out of its normal position with respect to the ones above and below, resulting in abnormal pressure on the spinal nerves and a denaturing or deforming of the spinal cord. 1994; A subluxation is a mechanical lesion that creates chronic sensory bed disturbance causing reflexes which alter the function of the efferent nervous system causing muscular and visceral dysfunction, i.e., those reflexes which hurt the body.

Tendon: Connective tissue which attaches muscle to cartilage, or muscle to bone.

Thoracic: Middle twelve vertebrae below the cervicals which support the ribs and great internal organs of the chest.

Viscera: Large internal organs.

Whiplash: An acute cervical sprain, usually resulting from a deceleration/acceleration, flexion/extension type of injury.

Appendix A— Exercises

Neck Stretches

Start with your head looking straight forward

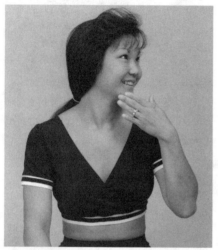

A *Gently rotate fully each direction*

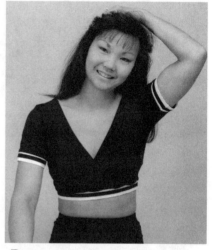

B *Gently stretch head to each side*

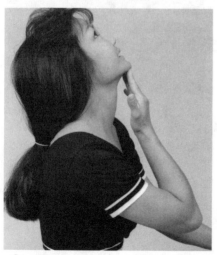

C *Gently push head back*

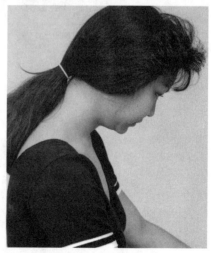

D *Gently stretch neck forward*

Neck range of motion stretches. In all except D, increased range of motion is attained by use of the hand to push or pull a little further.

Lower Back Stretches

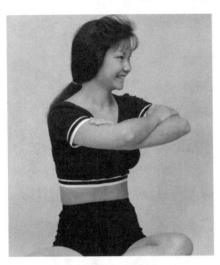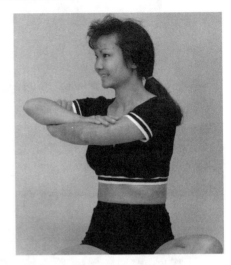

Lumbar Twists. Rotate fully to each side slowly and stretch each time. Keep your trunk straight as you twist your upper body.

Lower Back/Piriformis Stretch

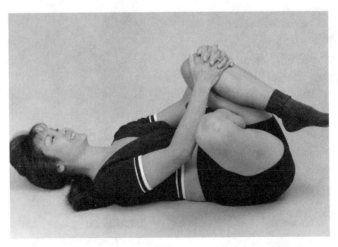

Pulling gently on the left leg will stretch the right piriformis to its maximum. Notice how the right foot is tucked into the lap.

Hamstring Stretch

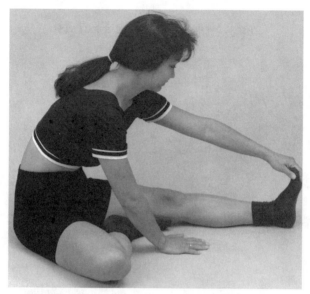

This is essential for relieving lower back pain. Notice how she keeps her back relatively straight.

Back/Paraspinal Muscles Stretch

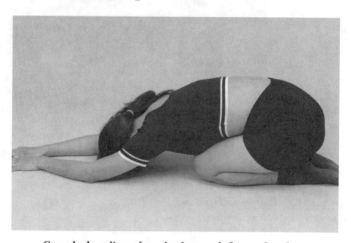

Start by kneeling, then slowly stretch forward and then back again.

Back Strengthening Exercises

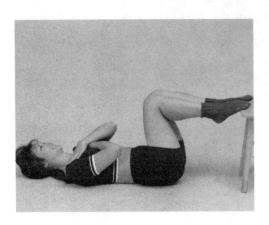

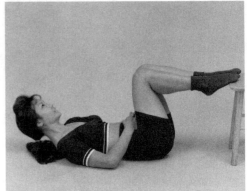

Crunch Type Sit-ups. Start with knees bent and the head and shoulders flat. Then raise up approximately 6" to 12", then lower. Use abdominal muscles only!

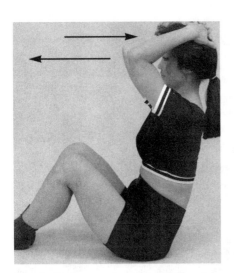

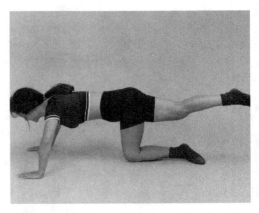

Kick-Back Exercises. Alternate raising legs. Do not extend legs above your buttocks or back.

Head resistance against arms pulling forward. Helps to strengthen neck/upper back muscles.

Resting/Sleeping Positions

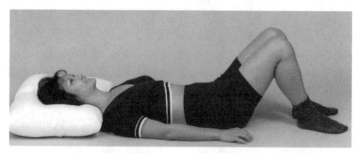

Correct Sleeping Position. Pillow has a neck roll which maintains a good cervical curve. Knees are bent and low back is flattened out to relieve pressure.

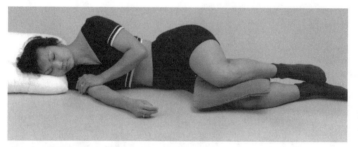

Correct Sleeping Position. Head should be lined up such that the neck and thoracic spines are straight. The pillow between the thighs will stabilize a sore back.

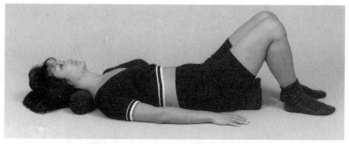

Lying on neck and low back supports. The neck roll maintains the cervical curve, while the triangular shaped wedge under the sacrum, flattens out the low back. This is a good position for lying on ice.

APPENDIX B
Anomalies of the Spine

Anomalies of the spine are simply areas in the spine which have abnormal structure, i.e., anatomical variants. These commonly occur as a result of congenital or hereditary factors. They may or may not be painful or dangerous. There are many fine books dedicated to an exhaustive listing of anomalies. The second chapter of Terry Yochum, D.C. and Lindsay Rowe, D.C.'s excellent text *Essentials of Skeletal Radiology* is one example.[92]

The information you are about to read is not quoted but is mostly derived from their book. We will limit our discussion to the most common and the most clinically significant types of anomalies, the ones you are most likely to encounter that cause pain.

(a) *Occipitalization of Atlas:* This occurs during the first few weeks of life when the vertebrae of the cervical spine separate and form. It can be viewed on a lateral cervical (side view of the neck) x-ray. It appears as if the atlas (C1) and the base of the skull are fused together. Clinically there should be no pain in childhood, but adults may develop degenerative joint disease if the lower cervical vertebrae move too much as a consequence of the fusion. The spinal cord may also become compressed at that level due to instability of a ligament known as the transverse ligament. This could cause severe neurological problems. The transverse ligament acts as a stabilizer where C1 sits on C2. Without this ligament the chiropractor could not adjust on C1 unless it is determined to be stable.

(b) *Posterior Ponticle:* A posterior ponticle of the atlas occurs in a small percentage of patients (approximately 15%). It is a calcification which forms a small bridge across the posterior arch and the body, or lateral masses of C1.

It may occur on one or both sides and is easily visualized on the lateral cervical x-ray. Its clinical significance lies in the fact that the vertebral artery, and possibly the first cranial nerve, pass through this opening. If the opening becomes constricted, it may temporarily diminish the flow of blood to the brain. Due to this, your doctor of chiropractic may decide not to manipulate the upper cervical spine; he or she would not adjust your neck in the traditional way. Instead, the Activator or a drop table technique such as Biophysics or Thompson may be used. (See the chapter entitled "*Different Techniques*")

(c)   *Down's Syndrome (Mongolism):* Down's Syndrome is due to a change in the 21st chromosome and occurs once in every 600 births. Patients at birth usually have a decreased diameter of the skull, slanting eyes, protruding tongue and a small flat nose. Mental retardation is also common with these patients, and there is an increased possibility of leukemia developing. The major point of clinical importance in these children is that there may be no transverse ligament of the atlas. This may occur in up to 20% of the patients. The chiropractor should take flexion/extension x-rays of the cervical spine in order to determine the stability of the upper cervical area. If there is stability, then the atlas adjustment may usually be performed safely if there are no other complications.

(d)   *Klippel Feil Syndrome:* People who have Klippel Feil Syndrome often have short, webbed necks, very little cervical range of motion and a low hairline. The reason patients cannot turn their head very much is because there are multiple blocked vertebrae in the lower cervical and upper thoracic spines. It is also possible that there may be other organ systems involved, such as the heart and lungs, the nervous system and genito-urinary system. In addition, there may also be rib deformity and/or Sprengel's deformity.

(e)   *Sprengel's Deformity:* Sprengel's Deformity is a congenital elevation of unknown origin of the shoulder blade (scapula) predominantly seen in females. One shoulder blade appears to be higher than the other, and there is a decreased ability of the arm to abduct (move away from the body, out to the side). Usually surgery is recommended between the ages of four and seven years. Although physical therapy is not helpful for the condition itself, chiropractic care and physical therapy may be beneficial after surgery.

(f)   *Cervical Rib:* The vertebrae of the thoracic spine, which starts at about the shoulder level, have ribs which extend out and around to the front of the chest. Here they join and form the sternum in front. The cervical vertebrae, of which there are seven, do not have ribs attached except in rare cases. A cervical rib usually attaches to the transverse process of the lowest cervical vertebrae, such as C5, C6, or C7.

This becomes clinically significant only if the brachial plexus (the bundle of nerves and blood vessels which exit the spine at the base of the neck and go down the arms) becomes compressed. This is especially true for people who droop their shoulders. If compression does occur, the patient may feel symptoms such as pain, numbness, coldness, or tingling into the arms or hands. This may be relieved by very specific chiropractic adjustments to the area.

I worked with a patient named Bill during my clinical rotation in chiropractic college who had a strange little osteophyte (outgrowth of bone) which hung down off the right transverse process of C7. It looked like a hanging stalactite and caused him much misery. We were able to control the symptoms by adjusting the vertebral rib beneath it down and away from the compressed area.

(g)   *Hemivertebrae:* Hemivertebrae are simply triangularly-shaped vertebrae that often appear in patients with structural scoliosis. The wedge is usually on the side of the vertebrae but occasionally is in the front or the back. Obviously this causes the spine to tilt in that direction.

(h)   *Schmoral's Nodes:* Schmoral's Nodes are small indentations in the endplates of the vertebrae due to degeneration of the disc. As the disc degenerates, the nucleus pulposus (the gelatinous center portion of the disc) protrudes through the bottom of the vertebrae above and the top of the vertebrae below. The nucleus cannot be compressed; it is like a contained ball of toothpaste.

When great forces are imposed on it, either the fibrous rings which surround it will break (herniated disc) or the vertebral end plate above or below it will be penetrated. The force may be post-trauma, degeneration, malignant tumors, sickle cell anemia, or other diseases which involve bone.

(i)   ***Spina Bifida Occulta and Vera:*** Spina bifida means there is a failure of the lamina in the back of the vertebrae to close completely, leaving the spinal cord somewhat exposed. When it is "occulta" it is a small opening and will not generally cause back pain. However, "spina bifida vera" usually has a large opening and will allow protrusion of the spinal cord. This may contribute to back pain as well as a spinal cord which is unprotected at this spinal level.

It may be discovered at birth upon examination of the newborn. There may be a small patch of hair over the spinal level, a dimple, or a lipoma (fatty tumor). There may be herniation of the spinal cord coverings or the entire spinal cord itself into the soft tissues. This has the effect of decreasing or destroying the nerves at that level and interfering with the normal development of the fetus. Clubbed feet, paralysis, tumors and problems with walking are all manifestations of this disease. Surgery may be inevitable.

(j)   ***Transitional Vertebrae:*** Recall that the spine is divided into distinct regions or segments. There are the skull, cervical region, thoracic region, lumbar region, sacrum and coccyx. Each region has vertebrae which are specifically designed for that area. The areas between these regions are known as transitional areas; the vertebrae here change their characteristics from one region to the next. Transitional vertebrae have the distinction of having characteristics of both spinal regions.

They are most commonly found in the lumbosacral region. For example, the fifth "lumbar" may look more like the sacrum, or the first "sacral segment" may appear as the last lumbar vertebra. The problem occurs when there is inappropriate fusion or lack of fusion in that particular segment. This may result in too little or too much motion in these areas. The result is that the other adjacent areas of the spine must compensate for this defect. There may be pain and the vertebrae may be predisposed to subluxate. A chiropractor will help to reestablish proper movement in these spinal areas with specific spinal adjustments.

(k) *Facet Tropism:* Facet tropism can occur in the lumbar area where one facet literally points in a different direction than the other. One facet joint may be vertical and the other may be horizontal. There may be pain in these regions. The chiropractor will probably adjust your low back differently on one side than the other.

(l) *"Knife Clasp" Syndrome:* Knife Clasp Syndrome occurs when the spinous process of the L5 vertebra is elongated, and there is a spina bifida of the first sacral segment. Pain occurs as the patient extends or arches the back, and the long spinous process contacts the soft tissues on the sacrum. Adjustments to the patient's low back should be done in flexion to relieve the symptoms. Ice may be applied when there is inflammation and if there are no contraindications for using ice.

(m) *Congenital Hip Dysplasia:* The hip is a "ball and socket joint" with the head of the femur being the ball and the acetabulum of the hip being the socket. Persons with congenital hip dysplasia usually have either a small femur head and/or a shallow or absent acetabulum. Due to these defects the femur may displace itself laterally to the side and ride up high. Surgery may be indicated to create a new hip socket.

There are many more anomalies of the spine and if you wish to read a more exhaustive study of each of the above listed subjects, I refer you to the text *Essentials of Skeletal Radiology* by Yochum and Rowe.

APPENDIX C

This appendix provides some suggestions on how to speed the healing process and avoid spinal problems.

1. Avoid rubbing, probing or poking recently adjusted areas.

2. Avoid sudden twists or turns beyond normal limits of motion, especially in the neck area.

3. Avoid extreme bending of the spine in any direction; avoid stretching, reaching or other overhead work. Be careful when brushing or shampooing your hair.

4. Avoid bending or stooping to pick up objects; instead, bend your knees to reduce lower back strain.

5. When lifting, keep your back straight, bend your knees and let the legs bear the strain. Hold the lifted object as close to your body as possible.

6. When bathing, sit rather than recline in the tub. If you are tired and want to relax, it's better to lie in bed.

7. Follow the exercises demonstrated elsewhere in the book; avoid activities which jar or stress neck and spine.

8. Be conscious of your posture: stand tall, sleep tall and THINK tall!

The following general guidelines will help you maintain good health.

1. Set aside a special time each day for mental and physical relaxation.

2. When sitting, choose a chair with firmness to hold your weight comfortably, then sit straight. Avoid soft, overstuffed furniture. Recliners should keep your back in a normal straight position.

3.   Cross your legs at the ankles only, not at the knees. Crossing at the knees could aggravate back conditions and interfere with blood circulation to the legs.

4.   Get plenty of sleep so the body can repair itself.

5.   Sleep on a firm mattress, not too hard or too soft, but firm enough to hold your body level while your shoulders and buttocks depress into the mattress.

6.   Pillows should not be too high or low. The best pillow supports your head so the neck vertebrae are level with the rest of your spine. Avoid using two pillows; never lie on a couch with your head on an armrest.

7.   Sleep on your back or side with legs flexed slightly, not drawn up tightly. Avoid sleeping on your stomach. Raise your head off the pillow to change positions.

8.   Get out of bed by turning on your side and swinging your legs off the bed, then push yourself into a sitting position with your arms, minimizing neck strain.

9.   Don't read or watch TV in bed, especially with your head propped at a sharp or strained angle.

10.   Don't sleep sitting in a chair or other cramped quarters; when it's time to sleep, lie down in bed.

When Using Ice

NEVER USE ICE OR HEAT WITHOUT CONSULTING YOUR PHYSICIAN.

1.   The proper use of ice is to constrict local blood vessels and help decrease and prevent inflammation of soft tissues. It also has an analgesic (pain-killing) effect and will reduce muscle spasm.

2.   Ice packs are usually not placed directly on the skin. Use a towel or shirt between the ice and your body for 20 minutes every two hours. **(DO NOT EXCEED 20 MINUTES CONTINUOUSLY).**

3.   Slush immersion of body parts such as feet, hands, etc. are done with 50% crushed ice and 50% water for up to 10 minutes (you may do shorter periods) every two hours. Here the skin is directly in contact with the water. For your comfort, you may try placing the body part in cool water and gradually adding ice, but extend treatment time to 20 minutes.

4.   Never use ice therapy if you:

   a)   have periperal vascular disease.

   b)   have a heart condition such as a past heart attack.

   c)   cannot sense a cold sensation on your skin.

   d)   have a hypersensitivity to cold.

   e)   have Rheumatoid Arthritis.

   f)   have been frostbitten previously in that area.

   g)   have a fear of cold and ice.

   h)   cannot remove the ice quickly and easily.

   i)   have not consulted your doctor.

IF YOU HAVE QUESTIONS ABOUT ANY PHASE OF YOUR HEALTH CARE, CONSULT YOUR CHIROPRACTOR.

APPENDIX D

In Chapter 6, I described some popular chiropractic techniques. If you want further information on any of these methods, please contact these chiropractors directly.

Activator Method
Dr. Arlan Fuhr
P.O. Box 80317
Phoenix, AZ 85060-0317
(602) 224-0220

Applied Spinal Biomechanical
Engineering
Dr. Ronald Aragona
1820 East Main Street
Waukesha, WI 53186
(800) 255-3202

B.E.S.T.
Dr. M.T. Morter, Jr.
101 Pleasant Ridge Lane
Rogers, AR 72756
(501) 636-1274

Bio-Cranial Technique
International
Bio-Cranial Academy
1620 South Boulevard,
Suite 2-A
Charlotte, NC 28203
(704) 331-0715

Chiropractic Biophysics
Dr. Donald Harrison
170 Yellow Creek Road, Suite D
Evanston, WY 82930
(800) 346-5146

Chiropractic Manipulative Reflex
Technique (CMRT)
SORSI Headquarters
P.O. Box 8245
Prairie Village, KS 66208
(913) 649-2750

Copes Scoliosis Total Recovery
System
2531 Toulon Drive
Baton Rouge, LA
(800) 726-8869

Directional Non-Force Technique
Dr. Christopher F. John
D.N.F.T. Seminars
256 South Robertson Boulevard,
Suite 1636
Beverly Hills, CA 90211
(310) 657-2338

Gonstead
P.O. Box 46
Mt. Horeb, WI 53572
(608) 437-5585

Logan Basic
Logan College of Chiropractic
Schoettler Road
Box 1065
Chesterfield, MO 63006
(314) 227-0903

Network
Dr. Donald Epstein
2431 Merrick Road
Bellmore, NY 11710
(516) 785-1236

Neural Organization Technique
(N.O.T.)
Carl A. Ferreri, D.C., Ph.C.
3850 Flatlands Ave.
Brooklyn, NY 11234
(718) 253-9702

Neuromuscular Reeducation™
Dr. Peter J. Levy
955 Tornoe Road
Santa Barbara, CA 93105
(805) 687-2111

N.U.C.C.A.
National Upper Cervical
Chiropractic Association
217 West 2nd Street
Monroe, MI 48161
(313) 241-5755

Orthospinology
Dr. J.K. Humber, Jr.
2620-F Cobb Parkway, South
Smyrna, GA 30080
(770) 952-5353

Pettibon Biomechanics Institute
Dr. Burl Pettibon
10529-C Lakeview Avenue, S.W.
Tacoma, WA 98499
(253) 265-2702

Pierce Results System
Dr. Walter Pierce, Jr.
195 S. Westmonte Drive, Suite L
Altamonte Springs, FL 32714
(407) 682-1880

Pierce-Stillwagon Technique
Dr. Glen Stillwagon
767 Dry Run Road
Monongahela, PA 15063
(724) 258-6506

Receptor-Tonus (Nimmo)
Dr. Sheila K. Laws
1210 North 24th Street
Quincy, IL 62301
(217) 223-6170

Sacro-Occipital Technique
SORSI Headquarters
P.O. Box 8245
Prairie Village, KS 66208
(913) 649-2750

Roy W. Sweat, D.C.
Atlas Orthogonist
3274 Buckeye Road, N.E.
Atlanta, GA 30341
(770) 952-5353

Thompson Technique
Dr. Terrence Brady
5687 Woodruff Avenue
Lakewood, CA 90713
(562) 866-8384

Toftness Technique
Dr. David Toftness
102 South Keller
Amery, WI 54001
(715) 268-7500

Total Body Modification (TBM)
Dr. Victor Frank
1907 East Foxmoor Circle
Sandy, UT 84092
(801) 571-2411

Vector Point Cranial Therapy
Dr. David G. Denton
1194 Pacific Street, Suite 201
San Luis Obispo, CA 93401
(805) 543-2211

If all else fails, here are some additional ways of locating a specific practitioner.

1. Call a local chiropractic college in your city.

2. Chambers of commerce can provide information.

3. Check the telephone directory under "Chiropractors" for doctors close to home or office.

4. In some cities a chiropractic directory service may be available by telephone. It probably only lists paid subscribers and is a form of advertising.

5. Newcomer services such as Welcome Wagon.

6. As brought to the attention of the American public in a supplement contained in the April, 1988, *Readers Digest*, "So a Chiropractor Is Really a Family Doctor." A referral can be requested from the national, state, or local chiropractic association, which will have a registry of members.

The National Directory of Chiropractic 1994–1995 is published by One Directory of Chiropractic, Inc., P.O. Box 10056, Olathe, KS 66051. Toll Free (800) 888-7914

Colleges of Chiropractic

Chiropractic will increase in popularity as people such as yourself become more familiar with its practices and potential. This will necessitate more and better trained chiropractors. If you are interested in finding out about a career in chiropractic and the training it requires, this list of chiropractic colleges in the United States and some other parts of the world is a starting point. Contact each college directly for specifics about their curriculum.

UNITED STATES

Cleveland Chiropractic College
6401 Rockhill Road
Kansas City, MO 64131
(816) 333-8230

Cleveland Chiropractic College
(L.A. Campus)
590 North Vermont Avenue
Los Angeles, CA 90004
(213) 660-6166
(800) 466-2252

Life College
1269 Barclay Circle
Marietta, GA 30060
(770) 426-2600
(800) 543-3348

Life Chiropractic College West
2005 Via Barrett
P.O. Box 367
San Lorenzo, CA 94580
(510) 276-9013
(800) 778-4476

Logan College of Chiropractic
1851 Schoettler Road
P.O. Box 1065
Chesterfield, MO 63006
(314) 227-2100

Los Angeles College
of Chiropractic
16200 East Amber Valley Drive
P.O. Box 1166
Whittier, CA 90609
(562) 947-8755
(800) 221-5222

National College of Chiropractic
200 East Roosevelt Road
Lombard, IL 60148
(630) 629-2000
(800) 826-NATL

New York Chiropractic College
2360 Route 89
P.O. Box 800
Seneca Falls, NY 13148-0800
(315) 568-3000
(800) 234-6922

Northwestern College
of Chiropractic
2501 West 84th Street
Bloomington, MN5543- 1599
(612) 888-4777

Palmer College of Chiropractic
1000 Brady Street
Davenport, IA 52803
(319) 326-9600
(800) 722-2586

Palmer College of
Chiropractic West
90 East Tasman Drive
San Jose, CA 95134
(408) 944-6000
(800) 442-4476

The Parker College
of Chiropractic
2500 Walnut Hill Lane
Dallas, TX 75229-5612
(214) 438-6932
(800) 438-6932

University of Bridgeport
College of Chiropractic
Bridgeport, CT 06601
(203) 576-4279
(888) 822-4476

Sherman College of
Straight Chiropractic
Springfield Road
P.O. Box 1452
Spartanburg, SC 29304
(864) 578-8770
(800) 849-8771

Texas Chiropractic College
5912 Spencer Highway
Pasadena, TX 77505
(281) 487-1170

Western States
Chiropractic College
2900 Northeast 132nd Avenue
Portland, OR 97230
(503) 256-3180

AUSTRALIA

Royal Melbourne Institute
of Technology (RMIT)
Department of Chiropractic
Osteopathy
Plenty Road
Bundoora, Victoria 3083
011-61-3-9468-2440

Macquarie University
Centre for Chiropractic
P.O. Box 178
Summerhill, N.S.W. 2130
011-61-2-850-9380
FAX 011-61-2-716-7114

CANADA

Université du Québec
à Trois-Rivières
3351 Boul des Forges
Trois-Rivières, Quebec G9A 5H7
(819) 376-5186

Canadian Memorial
Chiropractic College
1900 Bayview Avenue
Toronto, Ontario M4G 3E6
Canada
(416) 482-2340

ENGLAND

Anglo-European College
of Chiropractic
13-15 Parkwood Road
Bournemouth, Dorset BH5 2DF
England
(011) (44) 1202-43-6200

FRANCE

French Institute of Chiropractic
44 rue Duhesme
75018 Paris
France
(33) (1) 42-59-80-20

JAPAN

Chukyo School of Chiropractic
3-12-12 Meieki Nakamuraku
Nagoya 450
Japan

Japan Chiropractic College Center
Nagaoka Building 5F
5-13-2 Ginza Chou-Ku
Tokyo
Japan

Tokyo Chiropractic College
Murakami No. 3 Building
1-60-7 Minami-Otsuka
Toshima-Ku Tokyo
Japan

SOUTH AFRICA

Technikon Natal
P.O. Box 953
Durban 4000
Nattechnikon 6-20187
South Africa
(031) 225-2111

References

1. Originally published August 1957 Chiropractic Home, Vol. XXI, No. 8 and reported recently in *The Chiropractic Journal*, Vol. 8, No. 9, June 1994

2. Dr. Greg Johnson, personal communication, July 1994

3. D.D. Palmer, *THE SCIENCE, ART, AND PHILOSOPHY OF CHIROPRACTIC*, Portland, OR: Portland Printing House, 1910

4. J.F. Bourdillon, M.D. with E.A. Day in *Spinal Manipulation* (4th ed.), Norwalk, CT: Appleton & Lange, 1987, 5

5. Robert S. Mendelsohn, M.D., *Confessions of a Medical Heretic*, Chicago: Contemporary Books Inc., 1979

6. Charles B. Inlander, Lowell S. Levin and Ed Weiner, *Medicine on Trial: The Appalling Story of Medical Ineptitude and the Arrogance that Overlooks It*, New York: The People's Medical Society, published by Pantheon Books, 1988

7. Dr. Dan Murphy, personal communication

8. B. Wyke, Ph.D, "Articular Neurology and Manipulative Therapy," in R.M. Idezak, *ASPECTS OF MANIPULATIVE THERAPY*, London: Carlito Lincoln Institute of Health Science, 1980

9. Foster Hibbard, personal communication

10. Ruth Jackson, M.D., *THE CERVICAL SYNDROME*, Springfield, IL: Charles C. Thomas Co, 1977

11. H. Kamieth, *PATHOGENIC IMPORTANCE OF THE THORACIC IMPORTANCE OF THE VERTEBRAL COLUMN*, Arch. orthop.u.Unfall-Chir. 49:585-606 (No. 6) 1958 (in German) [Munich, Germany]

12. Charles Sallahian, D.C., "Reduction of a Scoliosis in an Adult Male Utilizing Specific Chiropractic Spinal Manipulation: A Case Report", *CHIROPRACTIC: THE JOURNAL OF CHIROPRACTIC RESEARCH AND CLINICAL INVESTIGATION*, Vol. 7, No. 2, July 1991, 42-45

13. Rene Cailliet, M.D., *SOFT TISSUE PAIN AND DISABILITY*, Philadelphia: A. Davis Co., 1977

14. Nikolai Bogduk, Ph.D. and Lance T. Twomey, Ph.D., *CLINICAL ANATOMY OF THE LUMBAR SPINE*, New York: Churchill Livingstone, 1987

15. Rene Cailliet, M.D., see note 13

16. Alf Breig, M.D., *ADVERSE MECHANICAL TENSION IN THE CENTRAL NERVOUS SYSTEM*, Stockholm: Almqvist & Wiksell International/New York: John Wiley and Sons, 1978

17. Bogduk and Twomey, see note 14

18. Stephen C. Waddell, D.C., Joseph S. Davidson, Ph.D., A. Dean Befus, Ph.D., Ronald D. Mathison, Ph.D., "Role for the Cervical Sympathetic Trunk in Regulating Anaphylactic and Endotoxic Shock," *JOURNAL OF MANUPULATIVE AND PHYSIOLOGICAL THERAPEUTICS*, Vol. 15, No. 1, 1992, 10-15

    Akio Sato, M.D., Ph.D., "The Reflex Effects of Spinal Somatic Nerve Stimulation on Visceral Function", *JOURNAL OF MANUPULATIVE AND PHYSIOLOGICAL THERAPEUTICS*, Vol. 15, No. 1, 1992, 5741

    James M. Allen, "The Effects of Chiropractic on the Immune System: A Review of the Literature", *CHIROPRACTIC JOURNAL OF AUSTRALIA*, Vol. 23, No. 4, December 1993, 132-135

19. Stanley Hoppenfield, M.D., *ORTHOPAEDIC NEUROLOGY—A DIAGNOSTIC GUIDE TO NEUROLOGICAL LEVELS*, Philadelphia: J.B. Lippincott Co., 1977

20. *MERCK MANUAL OF DIAGNOSIS AND THERAPY* (15th ed.), Rahway, NJ: Merck Sharp and Dohme Research Laboratories Division of Merck and Co. Inc. 1987

21. T.W. Meade, M.D. et al, *BRITISH MEDICAL JOURNAL*, 300:1431-37, 1990; "Proceedings of the Sixth Annual Conference on Research and Education," Paul Shekelle, M.D., M.P.H., RAND Corporation, 1991 (hereafter RAND Report); Pran Manga et al, Ontario Ministry of Health, "The Effectiveness and

Cost Effectiveness of Chiropractic Management of Low-Back Pain." 1993 (hereafter Manga Report)

22. Gary M. Franklin et. al. "Outcome of Lumbar Fusion in Washington State Workers' Compensation" *SPINE*, Vol. 19, No. 17, 1994, 1897-1904. Franklin also states that 67% of patients reported that back pain was worse and 55 % stated that quality of life was no better or worse than before surgery.

23. Stanley Bigos, M.D. and Michele Crites Battie, "Acute Care to Prevent Back Disability: Ten Years of Progress" *CLINCIAL ORPTHOPAEDICS AND RELATED RESEARCH*, Vol . 221, August 1987, 121 - 130

24. Robert O. Becker, M.D. and Gary Seldon, *THE BODY ELECTRIC*, New York: Morrow, 1986

25. J. Kraemer, D. Kolditz, and R. Gowin, "Water and Electrolyte Content of Human Intervertebral Discs under Variable Load," *SPINE*, Vol. 10, No. 1, 1985, 69-71

26. Donald Murphy, D.C., "Myofaschl Pain and Failed Back Surgery", *DYNAMIC CHIROPRACTIC*, Motion Palpation Institute, August, 2, 1991, 8

27. William Kirkaldy-Willis, *MANAGING LOW BACK PAIN*, (2nd ed.), New York: Churchill Livingstone, 1988; and H. Tilscher and M. Hanna, "Causes of Poor Results of Surgery in Low Back Pain," *MANUAL MEDICINE*, Vol. 5, No. 3, 1990, 110-114

28. Donald Murphy, "Scalene Trigger Points: The Great Imitators," *DYNAMIC CHIROPRACTIC*, Motion Palpation Institute, November 22, 1991

29. Janet Travell and David G. Simons, *MYOCSCIAL PAIN AND DYSFUNCTION: THE TRIGGER POINT MANUAL*, Baltimore: Williams and WiLkins, 1983

30. *MERCK MANUAL*, see note 20, 1258

31. T. Yamauchi, Y. Yamauchi, and K. Miura, "The Analgesic Effects of R.A. by Moving at Awakening and 'Sleeping Time,'" *PAIN* 1987; Suppl 4:S261

32. John A. McDougall, *M.D.*, *McDougall's Medicine, A Challenging Second Opinion*, Piscataway, NJ: New Century Publisher, Inc., 1985

33. Donald Murphy, D.C., "Shoulder Pain," *Dynamic Chiropractic*, Motion Palpation Institute, June 7, 1991

34. "Running Injuries", *Clinical Symopsia*, Vol. 39, No. 3, 1987, Ciba Geigy Corporation, 31. Also see Kirkaldy-Willis, note 27

35. Irvin Korr, Ph.D., *Collected papers of Irvin M. Korr*, American Academy of Osteopathy, 1979

36. Irvin Korr, Ph.D., see note 35

37. J.T. Freeman, "Posture in the Aging and Aged Body." *Journal of the American Medical Association*, Vol. 165, No. 7, 1957, 843-846

38. John Lennon, B.M., M.M., C. Norman Shealy, M.D., Roger K. Cady, M.D., William Matta, Ph.D., Richard Cox, Ph.D., and William F. Simpson, Ph.D., "Postural and Respiratory Modulation of Autonomic Function, Pain, and Health. " *American Journal of Pain Management*, Vol. 4, No. 1, 1994, 36-39

39. Ronald Pero, Ph.D. lecture in San Francisco, California, April 1985

40. James M. Allen, B.C.A., B.V.Sc., D.C., see note 18

41. Dan Murphy, D.C., D.A.B.C.O.,*Chiropractic Biophysics Level V. Posture and Health*, Pleasanton, CA, 1991

42. Dan Millman, *The Peaceful Warrior*, Tiburon, CA: H.J. Kramer, Inc., 1980

43. Raymond R. Brodeur, D.C., Ph.D. and Harry L. Wallace, D.C., "Cervical Spine Intervertebral Kinematics for Females Suffering from Headaches: A Preliminary Study," *Chiropractic: The Journal of Chiropractic Research and Clinical Investigation*, Vol. 8, No. 4, 1993, 73-77

44. Travels and Simons, see note 29

45. P.C . Brennan et al., "Enhanced Phagocytic Cell Respiratory Burst Induced by Spinal Manipulation: Potential Role of Substance P." *JOURNAL OF MANIPULATIVE AND PHYSIOLOGICAL THERAPEUTICS*, Vol.14, No.7, 1991, 399-408

46. R. Munroe-Ford, "Asthma Fight Falters as the Nation's Death Toll Mounts, " *Medical Forum in WEEKEND AUSTRALIAN*, January 4, 1992, 22

47. C.P. Van Schayct et al., "Bronchodilator Treatment in Moderate Asthma or Chronic Bronchitis: Continuous or on Demand? A Randomized Controlled Study" *BRITISH MEDICAL JOURNAL*, Vol. 303, 1991, 14261431

    M.R. Sears et al., "Regular Inhalated Beta-agonists Treatment in Bronchial Asthma, "*LANCET*, Vol. 336, 1990, 1391-1396

    W.O. Spitzer et al., "The Use of Beta-agonists and the Risk of Death and Near Death from Asthma," *New England Journal of Medicine*, Vol. 326, 1992, 501506

48. Dean H. Lines, D.C., "A Wholistic Approach to the Treatment of Bronchial Asthma in a Chiropractic Practice", *CHIROPRACTIC JOURNAL OF AUSTRALIA*, Vol. 23, No. 1, 1993, 4-8

    See also Niels Nilsson, D.C., M.D. and Bruno Christiansen, D.C., "Prognostic Factors in Bronchial Asthma in Chiropractic Practice", *JOURNAL OF THE AUSTRALIAN CHIROPRACTIC ASSOCIATION*, Vol. 18, No. 3, 1988, 1185-1187

49. H. Winsor, M.D., "Sympathetic Segmental Disturbances-ll. The Evidence of the Association in Dissected Cadavers of Visceral Diseases with Vertebrae Deformities of the Same Sympathetic Segments", *MEDICAL TIMES*, Vol. 49, November 1921, 1-7

    MANUAL OF OSTEOPATHIC PRACTICE (2nd ed.), London: Stoddard A. Hutchinson and Co, 1983, 16

    C. Masarsky and M. Weber, "Chiropractic Management of Chronic Obstructive Pulmonary Disease", *JOURNAL OF MANIPULATIVE AND PHYSIOLOGICAL THERAPEUTICS*, December 1988, 505-510

G. Melin and R. Harajula, "Lung Function in Relation to Thoracic Spinal Mobility and Kyphosis", *SCANDINAVIAN JOURNAL OF REHABILITATIVE MEDICINE*, Vol. 19, 1987, 89-102

W.D. Miller, D.O., *TREATMENT OF VISCERAL DISORDERS BY MANIPULATIVE THERAPY*, 1975

A. Howell, "The Influence of Osteopathic Manipulative Therapy in the Management of Chronic Obstructive Lung Disease", *JOURNAL OF THE AMERICAN OSTEOPATHIC ASSOCIATION.* 74, 1975, 757-760

Cited by Tedd Koren, D.C., in "Asthma, Emphysema, and Bronchitis", Philadelphia: Koren Publications, 1991

50. William A. Nelson, D.C., "Diabetes Mellitus: Two Case Reports," *CHIROPRACTIC TECHNIQUE*, Vol. 1, No. 2, May 1989

51. R.L. Dickinson, D.C., "Effects of Chiropractic Spinal Adjustments and Interferrential Therapy in the Restoration of Peripheral Circulatory Impairment in the Lower Extremities of Diabetics," *CHIROPRACTIC*, April, 1988

52. See notes 5 and 31

53. R.G. Yates, D.L. Lamping, N.L. Abram, C. Wright, "The Effects of Chiropractic Treatment on Blood Pressure and Anxiety: A Randomized Controlled Trial. "*JOURNAL OF MANIPULATIVE AND PHYSIOLOGICAL THERAPEUTICS*, Vol. 11, No. 6, 1988, 4848.

54. A.D. Miller, A REVIEW OF HYPERTENSION AND ITS MANAGEMENT BY OSTEOPATHIC MANIPULATIVE THERAPY, Academy of Applied Osteopathy, *1966 Yearbook*, 30-36.

M.E. McKnight and K.F.DeBoer, "Preliminary Study of Blood Pressure Changes in Normotensive Subjects Undergoing Chiropractic Care," *JOURNAL OF MANIPULATIVE AND PHYSIOLOGICAL THERAPEUTICS*, 11: 1988, 261-266.

G. Dulgar, D. Hill, A. Sirucek, and B. Davis, "Evidence for a Possible Anti-hypertensive Effect of Basic Technique Apex Contact Adjusting", *ACA JOURNAL OF CHIROPRACTIC*, 14: 1980, S97-S 102

T.A. Tran and J.D. Kirby, "The Effect of Upper Thoracic Adjustment Upon the Normal Physiology of the Heart", *ACA JOURNAL OF CHIROPRACTIC*, 11: 1977, 25-28 and 58-62

H . A. Blood, *MANIPULATIVE MANAGEMENT OF HYPERTENSION*, Academy of Applied Osteopathy, 1964 Yearbook, 189-195

All cited by Tedd Koren, D.C. in "Blood Pressure and Chiropractic", Philadelphia: Koren Publications, 1989

55. Mendelsohn, see note 5

56. Michael Schmidt, D.C., personal communication

57. Robert J. Goodman, D.C. and John S. Mosby, Jr., D.C., M.D., "Cessation of a Seizure Disorder," *CHIROPRACTIC: THE JOURNAL OF CHIROPRACTIC RESEARCH AND CLINICAL INVESTIGATION*, Vol. 6, No. 2, July 1990, 43-46

58. M.A. Harvey, R.J. Johns, V.A. McKusick, A.H. Owens, and R.S. Ross, "Syncope, Seizures, and other Episodic Disorders "in THE PRINCIPLES AND PRACTICE OF MEDICINE (22nd ed.), Appleton and Lange, 1988, 1032.

    G. Young, "Chiropractic Successes in Epileptic Conditions ", *ACA JOURNAL OF CHIROPRACTIC*, April 1982.

    Cited by Tedd Koren, D.C. in "Seizures, Epilepsy and Chiropractic", Philadelphia: Koren Publications, 1991

59. David E. Stude, D.C., "The Management of Symptoms Associated with Premenstrual Syndrome," *JOURNAL OF MANIPULATIVE AND PHYSIOLOGICAL THERAPEUTICS*, Vol. 14, No. 3, 1991, 209-215.

60. Mark A. Wittler, D.C., Chiropractic Approach to Premenstrual Syndrome (PMS)," *CHIROPRACTIC: The Journal of Chiropractic Research and Clinical Investigation*, Vol. 8, No. 2, 1992, 26-29

61. The following material is based on some suggestions of Phillip W. Harvey, Ph.D, R.D. in his *CLINICAL NUTRITION DESK REFERENCE* (3rd ed.), 1993

62. Pettybon, 1978

63. Meade et al, *BRITISH MEDICAL JOURNAL*, 300: 1990, 1431-37,;
    K.B. Jarvis, D.C., R.B. Phillips, D.C., Ph.D., E. K. Morris,
    J.D., M.B.A., "Cost per Case Comparison of Back Injury Claims
    of Chiropractic versus Medical Management of Conditions with
    Identical Diagnostic Codes, "*JOURNAL OF OCCUPATIONAL
    MEDICINE*, August, 1991; RAND study, 1991, Santa Monica,
    CA, 1993

    See also the Stano/Medstat Research; Manga; New Zealand;
    State of California Industrial Back Injury; and Nevada Workers'
    Compensation studies as summarized in *CALIFORNIA
    CHIROPRACTIC ASSOCIATION JOURNAL*, December 1993, 27-28

64. Chrisoula Eliopoulos, BSc, July Klein, MSc, My Khanh Phan,
    BSc, Brenda Knie, R.T., Mark Greenwald, M.D., David
    Chitayat, M.D., and Gideon Koren, M.D., "Hair
    Concentrations of Nicotine and Cotinine in Women and their
    Newborn Infants," *JOURNAL OF THE AMERICAN MEDICAL
    ASSOCIATION*, Vol. 271, No. 8, 1994, 621-623

65. H. Biederman, "Kinematic Imbalances due to Suboccipital
    Strain in Newborns," *JOURNAL OF MANUAL MEDICINE*, Vol. 6,
    1992, 151-156

66. Mark S. Gottlieb, "Neglected Spinal Cord, Brain Stem and
    Musculoskeletal Injuries Stemming from Birth Trauma, "
    JOURNAL OF MANIPULATIVE AND PHYSIOLOGICAL THERAPEUTICS,
    Vol. 16, No. 8, 1993, 537-543

67. Jennifer Brandon Peet, *CHIROPRACTIC PEDIATRIC AND PRENATAL
    REFERENCE MANUAL* (2nd ed.), Baby Adjusters, Inc. Publications,
    1992

68. W.M. Van Breda and J.M. Van Breda, "A Comparative Study of
    the Health Status of Children Raised under the Health Care
    Models of Chiropractic and Allopathic Medicine", *CRJ*,
    Summer 1989, 101-103. Quoted by Tedd Koren, D.C. in
    CHIROPRACTIC, BRINGING OUT THE BEST IN YOU, Philadelphia:
    Koren Publications, 1994

69. J.M. Giesen, D.B. Center and R.A. Leach, "An Evaluation of
    Chiropractic Manipulation as a Treatment of Hyperactivity in

Children", *Journal of Manipulative and Physiological Therapeutics*, Vol. 12, October 1989, 353-363.

E.V. Walton, "Chiropractic Effectiveness with Emotional, Learning and Behavioral Impairments" *ICA Review*, Vol. 29, September 1975, 2-5, 21-22.

C.J. Phillips, "Case Study: The Effect of Utilizing Spinal Manipulation and Craniosacral Therapy as the Treatment Approach for Attention Deficit-Hyperactivity Disorder" in *Proceedings of the National Conference on Chiropractic and Pediatrics*, 1991, 57-74

Quoted by Tedd Koren, D.C. in *Chiropractic, Bringing Out the Best in You*, Philadelphia: Koren Publications, 1994

70. Lennon, see note 38 and Sato, note 18

71. Dr. Jan Corwin, personal communication

72. Anthony Lauro, D.C. and Brian Mouch, D.C., "Chiropractic Effects on Athletic Ability. "*Chiropractic: Journal of Chiropractic Research & Clinical Investigation*. Vol. 6, No. 4, 1991, 84-87

73. Ben Hogan with Herbert Warren Wind and Anthony Ravielli, *Ben Hogan's Five Lessons: The Modern Fundamentals of Golf*, A.S. Barnes and Co., 1957

74. Thomas C. Deters, D.C. and Jeff Everson, L.P.T., "The Hows and Whys of Back Pain," *Joe Weider's Muscle and Fitness*, March 1992, p.229, reprinted by permission

75. Dr. Ronald Fritz, personal communication

76. Allan G.J. Terrett, "Cerebral Dysfunction: A Theory to Explain Some of the Effects of Chiropractic Manipulation," *Chiropractic Technique*, Vol. 5, No. 4, 1993, 168-173

77. Greg Gilman, O.D. and John Bergstrand, D.C., "Visual Recovery Following Chiropractic Intervention," *Journal of Behavioral Optometry*, Vol. 1 No. 3, 1990, 73-74; Thomas J. Wood, M.D., ''Upper Cervical Adjustments may Improve Mental Function," *Journal of Manual Medicine*, Vol. 6, 1992, 215-216

78. J. Cyriax, *TEXTBOOK OF ORTHOPEDIC MEDICINE, VOLUME 1: DIAGNOSIS OF SOFT TISSUE LESIONS,* London: Balliere Tindall, 1982

79. "M.D.s Cervical Manipulation Causes Woman's Stroke ", *DYNAMIC CHIROPRACTIC,* Motion Palpation Institute, December 20, 1991, 33

80. Teri K. Novak, D. C., R. H. D., "Craniomandibular Dysfunction and TMJ Syndrome", *CALIFORNIA CHIROPRACTIC JOURNAL,* Vol. 16, No. 4, April 1991, 38

81. *MERCK MANUAL* and *McDOUGALL'S MEDICINE*

82. James Robbins, *DIET FOR A NEW AMERICA,* Walpole, MA: Stillpoint Publishing, 1987

83. John A. McDougall, note 32

84. P. Manga et al, see note 21

85. Jarvis et al., see note 63

86. Manga Report, State of California Industrial Back Injury Study, British Medical Research Council Study, Rand Study, Nevada Workers' Compensation Study, and Stano/ Medstat Research, see note 63

87. Scott Donkin, D.C., *SITTING ON THE JOB*

88. *SPINE,* Vol. 16, No. 10, 1991

89. Dr. Kirby Landis, personal communication

90. Ronald Pero, Ph.D., "Common Diagnostic and Therapeutic Procedures of the Lumbosacral Spine, The North American Spine Society's Ad Hoc Committee on Diagnostic and Therapeutic Proceedures," pp. 1161-1167

91. *DORLAND'S MEDICAL DICTIONARY—SHORTER EDITION,* Philadelphia: W.B. Saunders Company, 1980, 3

92. Terry Yochum D.C. and Lindsay Rowe, D.C., *ESSENTIALS OF SKELETAL RADIOLOGY,* Baltimore: Williams & Wilkins, 1987

Information for the Medical Complication Comparison page taken from the following sources:

THE CHIROPRACTIC REPORT, May 1994 ; Vol. 8, No. 3: 1-6;   Editor: David Chapman-Smith, LL.B. (Hons.), FICC (Hon).

"Postoperative brainstem and cerebellar infarcts" in *NEUROLOGY* March 1993; Vol. 43: 471-477, by B. Tettenborn, MD; L.R. Caplan, MD; M.A. Sloan, MD; C.J. Estol, MD; M.S. Pessin, MD; L.D. DeWitt, MD; C. Haley, MD; and T.R. Price, MD.

"A randomized trial of intravenous heparin in conjunction with Anistreplase(Anisoylated Plasminogen Streptokinase Activator Complex) in acute myocardial infarction: The Duke University clinical cardiology study (DUCCS) 1" in *Journal of the American College of Cardiology* January 1994; Vol 23, No 1: 11-18, by C. O'Connor, MD, FACC; R. Meese, MD, FACC; R. Carney, MD, FACC; J. Smith, MD, FACC; E. Conn, MD, FACC; J. Burks, MD, FACC; C. Hartman, MD, FACC; S. Roark, MD, FACC; N. Shadoff, MD, FACC; M. Heard III, MD, FACC; B. Mittler, MD, FACC; G. Collins, MD, FACC; F. Navetta, MD, FACC; J. Leimberger, PhD; K. Lee, PhD and R. Califf, MD, FACC.

"Clinical importance of thrombocytopenia occuring in the hospital phase after administration of thrombolytic therapy for acute myocardial infarction" in Journal of the American College of Cardiology,   March, 1994; Vol 23, No 4: 891-898, by R. Harrington, MD; D. Sane, MD; R. Califf, MD, FACC; C. Sigmon, MA; C. Abbottsmith, MD, FACC; R. Candela, MD, FACC; K. Lee, PhD and E. Topol, MD, FACC.

"Aspirin and hemorrhagic stroke", (Letter), in *STROKE,* 1991; Vol 22, No. 9: 1213-1214, by N. Mayo, MD; A. Levy, BSc and M. Goldberg, MSc.

"Basilar artery embolism after surgery under general anesthesia: A case report", in *NEUROLOGY,* September, 1993; Vol 43: 1856, by C. Miller Fisher, M.D.

Dr. Robert Roberts, Baylor University Medical School, (personal communication, September, 1994,)

Index

FURTHER INFORMATION

One of the challenges which faces an author of a book like this is the inclusion of the continual flow of new information which may be valuable to the reader. The following important studies were not included in the text of this book and are presented here:

A.I.D.S.

A small pilot study on how specific chiropractic adjustments would affect HIV positive patients was published in 1994. The results showed those in the adjusted group experienced a 48% increase in CD4 cell levels (immune system), and those who were not adjusted (the control group), experienced a 7.96% decline in the CD4 cell levels. The article went on to say that they were recommending a large study be conducted since there was such a positive response.

This is a very important study since we are looking for any way to fight A.I.D.S. Since chiropractic care has already been shown to help the immune system, someone with H.I.V should seek a good chiropractor as soon as possible. It may not cure, but there is a possibility it can help **(Selano, D.C., Jeffrey L., Hightower, D.C. Brett C., Pfleger, Ph.D., Bruce, Collins, D.C., Karen Freeley, Grostic, D.C., John, "The effects of specific upper cervical adjustments on the CD4 counts of HIV positive patients."** *Chiropractic Research Journal,* **Vol 3: Number 1, 1994: pp 32-39).**

LOW BACK PAIN

In December, 1994, the Agency for Health Care Policy and Research (AHCPR) of the U.S. Department of Health and Human Services of the Federal Government of the United States recommended that spinal manipulation, usually conducted by Doctors of Chiropractic, is the best treatment for acute low back problems in adults. They also stated this type of conservative care should be pursued before surgery and that most prescription drugs such as oral steroids, colchicine and antidepressants were not recommended.

This reflects what chiropractors and their patients have been saying for the last 100 or more years. Chiropractic care gets results without the use of harmful drugs or surgery in all but the very worst cases. If you have a back problem, you should see a chiropractor first, or at least before you are subject to invasive medical therapies which are often useless at best and harmful at worst.

While you may first visit the chiropractor for your low back pain, keep in mind that most of us do not limit our practice to sore backs. In fact, as pointed out in this book, chiropractic care has been shown to help many other health problems.

MEDICAL ERRORS

A special communication was released in the December, 1994 issue of the *Journal of the American Medical Association* which discussed the large number of iatrogenic (physician caused) injuries and deaths which occur every year. The article estimated that 180,000 people die each year from medical intervention and a high percentage of these are medical errors. In fact, autopsy studies have shown a missed diagnosis was the cause of death in 35% to 40% of the cases. They say this is the equivalent of three jumbo-jet crashes every two days. Obviously this would be completely unacceptable in the transportation industry, but for some reason we have allowed it to continue in the medical field **(Leape, M.D., Lucian L., "Special Communication: Error in medicine;" *JAMA*, 1994; Vol 272: No 23; December 21, 1994, p. 1851-1857).**

A story which ran in the January 9, 1995 *U.S. News & World Report*, stated there was concern within the Federal Drug Administration over the side effects of several drugs prescribed for heart disease, cancer, arthritis and infections. The article estimated that up to two million people are hospitalized and 140,000 die each year from side effects or reactions to prescription drugs. The report also warned against halting any prescription medication without consulting a medical doctor.

These above reports are not meant to discredit anyone in the medical profession, but it is included as a warning to the consumer. Most, if not all, drugs and medical procedures have some adverse side effects and you need to question your medical doctor concerning all the associated risks.

SCOLIOSIS

A new bracing system that uses dynamic air pressure as a vectored force against an abnormally curved spine has been developed by Arthur Copes, PhD., Orthotist, of Baton Rouge, Louisiana. Dr. Copes works in conjunction with chiropractors to produce seemingly miraculous corrections of curvature of the spine (scoliosis) without surgery.

His patients have ranged in age from 8 to 65 years old, some with spinal curves over 40 degrees which responded to treatment. The cost is typically less than 25% of the costs of standard medical/surgical intervention. As of this writing, over 200 insurance carriers are covering part—if not all—of the costs associated with this form of scoliosis treatment.

About the Author
Dr. Michael Gazdar

Dr. Gazdar is a 1989 graduate of Life Chiropractic College West in San Lorenzo, California and is currently on the faculty as a part-time instructor in Chiropractic Technique. He maintains a full-time practice in Walnut Creek, California and often instructs weekend seminars for students and post-graduate chiropractors. He has lectured on chiropractic in Japan, Washington and New York.

In 1995, Dr. Gazdar received the prestigious "Alumni of the Year" award from Life West Chiropractic College.

Dr. Gazdar is an avid sports enthusiast. He runs, bicycles, and lifts weights daily to maintain fitness. He plays golf (previously a teaching professional), competitive softball, and is also a scuba diver and private pilot. Because of his sports background, Dr. Gazdar treats many serious athletes at different sporting events. In 1994, he completed studies to earn his Certified Chiropractic Sports Physician (C.C.S.P.), credential. This post-graduate training is essential for treating elite amateur and professional athletes.

Dr. Gazdar has lived in the San Francisco Bay Area all his life. He graduated from Richmond High School in 1976, attended Diablo Valley College, and earned a B.A. Degree in psychology from U.C. Berkeley in 1984. He also did Master's work in clinical psychology at Cal State, Hayward. He and his wife, Teri, have been married since 1991. They had their first baby, Christian Michael in April, 1994, and their second, Brandon Michael in June, 1996. They share their home with three cats—Smokey, Snow Flake and Garfield.

NOTES

NOTES

NOTES

NOTES

NOTES